Ulcerative Colitis Cookbook

Discover How To Relieve The Symptoms Of Ulcerative Colitis And Prevent Complications With Diet And 100 Healthy Recipes

Zoey Breana Rimmer

TABLE OF CONTENTS

Introduction

"Before starting I want to thank you for purchasing this book. I really hope this book will help you to relieve the symptoms of ulcerative colitis and prevent complications. I would love to receive your feedback with a review on Amazon when you finish. Enjoy the reading."

I am going to address this book to all the ones that suffer from ulcerative colitis. In a growing number of families at least one member is affected by this disease, some since they were children while others since later in life.

In this book, I decided to draw on literature about ulcerative colitis so that everyone who has just found out that they suffer from it or who has relatives who suffer from it can understand better what it is all about. Specifically I will cover topics such as the symptoms and causes that cause the disease. These are not yet fully known to modern medicine but I will try to give an answer based on medical sources that have treated me over the years.

In the second chapter instead I will focus on the impact that ulcerative colitis has on the immune system and on our health in general. To do this, I will draw on my personal experience.

Colitis is in fact a disease that can have serious consequences, particularly when of bacterial origin. In these cases, the particularly weakened patient can develop what is known as hemolytic-uremic syndrome, which can lead to kidney failure and septic shock.

Awareness is the first thing that enables individuals to act responsibly and in the right measure.

As everyone knows, ulcerative colitis requires not only pharmacological but also dietary treatment. Over the years, patients try a number of different kinds of food, from native to exotic, but many of them are harmful for those suffering from ulcerative colitis. So I will try to mention all the foods that you should not eat and those that are not related to the aggravation of colitis.

The goal of this chapter is to make people aware of the fact that a healthy and controlled diet can help the body in any situation, both in healthy people and in people with diseases. Thanks to the experience of the ones who surround me and the dieticians I have read about over the years, you can start right away on a balanced diet that is in line with your health condition. However, I recommend that you consult your doctor or dietician (who I am sure will confirm what you find out in the text).

Finally, chapter four includes 100 recipes of foods that are not harmful for most people suffering from ulcerative colitis so that you can immediately start preparing dishes that will not aggravate your health conditions and avoid those that can worsen them.

With that said, enjoy your reading!

Chapter 1: Everything you need to know about Ulcerative Colitis

1.1 What is Ulcerative Colitis?

It is important to have a helpful source for exploring and learning the things you are wondering about. This is not just for those who have been diagnosed with Ulcerative Colitis condition. This book is also for anyone that cares about someone with this condition or just wants to learn and help others. In this book, you will read about the Ulcerative Colitis condition. What it represents and what are the symptoms? Is there any known cause of this disease? Or are there only suggestions and thoughts from the scientists and doctors on what causes this condition. This disease can be very serious. But, also, it can have only mild symptoms. It affects our immune system in a very odd way. People with this disease are very limited when it comes to food and that is why it is important to explore any food that can make you feel better. Most of the food can trigger the condition and make the symptoms even worse than they already are. So, to manage Ulcerative Colitis you have to have a diet plan. There are things that you can eat that won't irritate the disease and it is best for you if you stick to the right diet. Some foods can even make the condition more bearable and for that matter, you should learn what foods can make that happen. Also, you can learn a lot about every beneficial nutrient that you can consume and better the condition. And because it is all part of our digestive system, it is important to know what will be easier to digest and what can cause a bigger problem.

Ulcerative Colitis is a gastrointestinal disease and an inflammatory bowel disease. It is a long-term condition, where the colon and the rectum become inflamed. It causes inflammation and ulcers in your digestive tract. Ulcerative colitis affects the innermost lining of your large intestine and rectum. An ulcer is a sore break in the skin, or on the inside lining of the body. This disease usually happens when your immune system makes a mistake. Ulcerative Colitis is thought to be an autoimmune condition. As a rule, our immune system attacks the invaders in our body, like the common cold. But, if you have Ulcerative colitis, the immune system thinks that food, the cells that line your colon, and good gut bacteria are the intruders. The white blood cells that generally protect our body, now attack the lining of our colon. That causes inflammation and ulcers. What exactly causes the immune system to behave in this particular way is still unclear. The severity of this disease depends on the amount of inflammation and the place where it is. In every person, it's a little different. You could have a very mild inflammation on the entire colon, which is a large area, or you could have a severe inflammation on a small area, like the rectum. This disease can be very serious for some patients. It starts in the rectum and extends proximally in a continuous manner, usually, through the entire colon. More often, ulcerative colitis is chronic with repeated exacerbations and remissions. Not being careful can lead to even bigger and more serious health problems. And, there are ways for this condition to be treated at home. But, only if the flare-ups are mild. Although, more severe flare-ups need to be treated in a hospital for reducing the risk of more serious and dangerous complications. Somehow, this disease is more common for the Jewish people. And the reason for that is unknown. Both women and men are equally able to get affected by Ulcerative Colitis. There are no rules about this condition. It can happen to anyone to get affected.

It affects the overall feeling of well-being too and it is important to feel well and good about yourself no matter what. Usually, knowing that other people have similar experiences can provide comfort, and the fact that you are not alone can change a lot for the better. Even if you are not the one diagnosed with Ulcerative Colitis, it is only natural to worry about your loved ones. And wanting to know about what they are going through while having this disease and learning about it, you might be able to understand them. And that can be very helpful to them. A book like this can help you learn about all the aspects and challenges of living with Ulcerative Colitis. It can also be helpful if you are newly diagnosed, or even if you have had it for years. The main thing and the most important one is to know all the facts about Ulcerative Colitis disease so that you know a better way to handle it. You should know all the things that are associated with this condition so that living with it won't be so bad.

In addition to this, I have put together some helpful recipes, since the struggle on what to eat while having Ulcerative Colitis is big. A healthy diet is a major thing in our life. It can better our mental health too, which is important. What you eat and consume has a big affection on our life. You should be aware of the fact that eating healthy and caring about your body and your mental health can drastically change your life and make it better. It is really important to keep a good diet. Your diet can make you function properly and have more energy. Keeping a positive mindset during difficult times won't make things any easier, but it is important to know that things will be better. It is hard enough living with a chronic condition, so leave all the negativity behind. You should always be grateful for what you have and for how far you have come. Having positive energy can make things feel better. And sometimes you have to motivate yourself to be better. Eating healthy, staying hydrated, and keeping a positive attitude can make living with this condition a little less exhausting.

I am hoping that the things you already read and the things that you are going to read in the next pages can help and that it can make the whole situation a little brighter. Sanguinely, you will find this book supportive and full of useful facts about the Ulcerative Colitis condition.

1.2 What are the main symptoms?

If you have this disease, you can notice that when symptoms are worse there is a pattern of flare-ups. Sometimes, during times of remission, you might have little too exactly no symptoms. The purpose of therapy and treatment is to remain in remission as long as possible, meaning more years.

Most of the people that are diagnosed with Ulcerative Colitis have light symptoms. However, there are people who have more serious symptoms. Ulcerative Colitis can cause many problems. Such as arthritis, eye inflammation, liver disease, and osteoporosis.

It is unknown why problems like this occur outside the colon. Some think that it is a result of inflammation triggered by the immune system. And most of the problems go away when the disease is treated.

Ulcerative colitis does not have an age range. It can happen to anyone. Although, it usually starts between the age of 15 and 30. As well as, between the age of 50 and 70. It can affect men and women. However, there is a study that people of particular ethnicities are more likely to get this disease.

There is more than one type of Ulcerative Colitis. It often depends on where it is in your body.

Ulcerative proctitis is the lightest and the mildest form of this disease. It's in the rectum. That's the part of your colon closest to your anus and the only sign of this disease might be rectal bleeding.

Another type is Proctosigmoiditis. What happens in your rectum and the lower end of your colon, also known as the sigmoid colon. Here, the symptoms are more serious. Proctosigmoiditis can cause rectal bleeding, rectal pain, diarrhea, and cramp. While this is a lifelong condition, there is some medication that can help you treat the symptoms. Although, some cases require surgery. Because complications can range from rectal bleeding to an even higher risk of colon cancer.

Left-sided colitis is yet another type. This one causes cramps on the left side of your stomach. It also causes diarrhea and inflammation from Pancolitis usually affects the entire colon. This can also cause diarrhea, cramps, and weight loss.

Acute severe ulcerative colitis is a very rare type. It affects the entire colon and causes severe pain, fever, bleeding and also, diarrhea.

If you already have Ulcerative Colitis, chances are big that you might develop further health problems. And often, more serious and dangerous conditions.

For example, people that are diagnosed with Ulcerative Colitis are at an increased risk of developing osteoporosis. Osteoporosis is a disease where the bones become weak and are more likely to fracture. This disease is not caused by Ulcerative Colitis directly, but it can develop as a side effect of the prolonged use of some medications that are used for treatment. Osteoporosis can also be caused by the dietary changes someone with Ulcerative Colitis may take. Because, avoiding dairy products can lower the level of calcium, however, dairy products are likely to trigger Ulcerative

Colitis symptoms. So, in that matter, you should probably take medication or supplements of vitamin D and calcium, which will strengthen your bones.

As said previously, children can also get affected by the Ulcerative Colitis condition. And some of the medications that are used for its treatment can affect growth and delay puberty. In addition to this, young people and children should have their body weight and height measured more regularly. This kind of check should be done every 3 to 12 months, it depends on the person's age and the treatment they are having as well as the severity of the symptoms they are having.

Furthermore, there is another rare but very serious complication of severe Ulcerative Colitis. Toxic megacolon is when inflammation in the colon causes gas to become trapped, emerging in the colon becoming swollen and enlarged. This can be very dangerous because it can cause the colon to split and cause infection in the blood. Some of the symptoms of toxic megacolon include pain in the abdominal area, a rapid heart rate, and high temperature or fever. The toxic megacolon condition can be treated with antibiotics, some fluids, and steroids that are given directly into a vein. In some cases, medications are not able to improve the condition quickly and because of that, surgical removal of the colon may be needed. That is why it is important to treat the Ulcerative Colitis symptoms before they become severe. It can help prevent toxic megacolon.

Although both men and women can get affected by Ulcerative Colitis condition, some studies have shown that it can affect both genders differently. Hormones and other sex-specific characteristics may play a big role in how some diseases, such as this one, affect men differently than women. In some cases, the difference of affection can be related to how men and women receive treatment for the illness.

Women who are diagnosed with Ulcerative Colitis are more likely to trigger the symptoms because of menstruation. Ulcerative Colitis may contribute to sexual dysfunction and menstrual cramps. Moreover, hormonal changes that occur during pregnancy and menstruation can trigger Ulcerative Colitis symptoms and can cause problems such as body image issues and yeast infection. The menstrual period is likely to aggravate the Ulcerative Colitis condition. Symptoms such as more gas or bloating, increased frequency of bowel movements, increased abdominal pain and diarrhea can get worse and during the menstrual period, according to some women. Experiencing more symptoms during menstruation may be caused by hormonal changes. Because, during the period women produce more hormone-like compounds, also known as prostaglandins, which can cause increased contractions of the smooth muscles in the colon. And this is the cause of more gastrointestinal problems. Some of them include diarrhea and abdominal cramps. Sometimes, abdominal cramps can get really unbearable. However, these symptoms do not necessarily lead to increased inflammation or a flare.

There is a medication used for the treatment of Ulcerative Colitis that can cause yeast infection. Medication such as immune-suppressing drugs are used very commonly for the treatment of Ulcerative Colitis and it can lead to vaginal yeast infection.

Another thing that is more likely a problem in women is body image. Mostly, women who have had an ostomy or surgery may be more affected. Some might also be worried about weight variation. Because there are medications that are used for this treatment that can lead to weight gain. And also there are medications used that can cause weight loss, which is more likely. This kind of problem can provide an increased risk of depression and anxiety, as well. It can also make some women discouraged from being sexually intimate. The way we think about our bodies can have a big impact on how we feel about sexual attractiveness. If any of these things concern you, you should talk to a specialist and work on the problem.

Another disease that men are at higher risk of getting affected by is colorectal cancer. Patients affected by this disease are encouraged to get screened regularly, because colorectal cancer can be treatable, if found early, of course.

Some men can also experience erectile dysfunction or have a lower level of sexual desire. There is a treatment for this, though.

Still, it is not understood why there are differences between men and women diagnosed with Ulcerative Colitis condition. Some studies suggest that genetics, lifestyle, environmental factors, as well as, hormones might be an actual valid reasons why all this happens.

Although a cure for Ulcerative Colitis is not found yet, there is a good deal of medications and treatments that are available to help relieve the symptoms and keep the triggers under control. Medications and treatment can be useful and they can allow the patients to have an active and more normal life.

Symptoms can be treated and the medications are working most of the time. However, in some cases, medication just is not able to relieve the Ulcerative Colitis symptoms and when this happens, surgery is needed. If surgery proceeds, the rectum or the colon are going to be removed, depends on where the Ulcerative Colitis is severe. This type of surgery will allow you to have bowel movements. Some studies have shown that 25 to 40 percent of the people diagnosed with Ulcerative Colitis eventually require surgery and have their colon or rectum removed.

However, if the symptoms from the Ulcerative Colitis condition are mild, surgery is not needed.

There is a possibility that complications can occur after the surgery is done. Some of which can cause more frequent and watery bowel movements. Inflammation of the pouch and blockage of the bowel obstruction from the internal scar tissues can also be caused by the surgery that is done.

Surgery is suggested if the medications and other treatments are not able to control the inflammation and ulcers right. However, surgery is also required if you get an emergency complication of the Ulcerative Colitis condition such as tears in the colon or severe bleeding.

1.3 What are the main causes behind the condition?

The exact reason why Ulcerative Colitis appears is not known. It was suspected that diet and stress were the cause, but lately, it's thought that this just aggravates the disease, however, it is not the main cause.

An immune system malfunction may be one of the possible causes. When the immune system tries to fight off an invader, a bacterium, or a virus, there's a response from the immune system that is odd. The immune system attacks the cells in the digestive tract, as well. That is abnormal feedback that the immune system gives during this condition.

Ulcerative Colitis can also be inherited. This disease is more common in people who already have someone in the family with the same condition. But, that's not the only way to get it. Also, there are people with ulcerative colitis that don't have any family member affected by this disease.

Where you live and how you live also seem to affect your chances of developing ulcerative colitis. This means that environmental factors are important, as well. In urban areas of northern parts of western Europe and America, this condition is more common. Air pollution, medication, and certain diets have also been studied. So far, nothing really proves the real cause of this disease. However, reduced exposure to bacteria may be an important factor that causes Ulcerative Colitis.

So, basically, the three factors that contribute to the development of Ulcerative Colitis disease are immune system response, genetics, and environmental factors. The immune system not responding properly to the intestinal tract results in inflammation and this causes Ulcerative Colitis. Moreover, in a way genetics predicts that there is a possibility that the disease will occur and that it can be inherited. The environmental factors are not absolutely identified. We still do not know what environmental factors are actually influencing and triggering the symptoms, however, something does trigger them and it initiates a harmful immune response in the intestines.

Ulcerative Colitis disease is unpredictable. No one can know how it will and how it can affect the diagnosed person. Because the disease is different for everyone. It can be similar to some people, but often, it is more likely to be different. Some people experience mild symptoms and the disease is not that bad. But, the ones that have the severe symptoms are experiencing the more painful and more serious part of the Ulcerative Colitis disease. It is not known what causes the disease to be more intense for some people.

Ulcerative Colitis is not caused by something the person diagnosed with it did. You cannot catch it from someone else, it is not contagious. This disease is not caused by something you consumed. It is not a result of something you ate or something you drank. It can be developed from a stressful and overwhelming lifestyle. Anyone can be affected by Ulcerative Colitis condition. This condition can affect both men and women equally as I said previously. People of any age can be diagnosed with Ulcerative Colitis. It can affect children and young people as well as adults and elderly people. Ethnicity does not play any role in this, too. Neither does race. Literally, anyone can get affected by a disease and still not know the cause of why it happened.

There are many suggestions on what possible causes could be. Some of them include food sensitivity. This can cause symptoms if the diagnosed person eats trigger foods, such as dried fruit or gluten and dairy.

Another suggestion is bacteria that produce toxins and can irritate the lining of the colon, so this may also be a cause. In addition to this, some viruses are also able to trigger inflammation.

There is also a possibility that some medications can be yet another cause for Ulcerative Colitis. Medications such as ibuprofen and aspirin can also irritate the lining of the colon. Into the bargain, severe reactions to antibiotics are also something that is considered a cause.

However, these are only suggestions. Although there is a possibility that each of these suggestions can be an actual cause, it is now proven. It is still unclear and unknown what is the real cause behind the Ulcerative Colitis condition.

Chapter 2: Autoimmune condition and general health

The immune system is the key to our survival. Without an immune system, the body could be easily attacked by viruses, bacteria, parasites, and more. The immune system is what keeps the body safe and protected from all toxic materials. The immune system actually represents a network of cells and tissues that is spread throughout the whole body and it involves many types of organs and proteins. The immune system consists of many parts. All the parts work together to defend the body against all the toxic materials attacking it. The network of cells and tissues is always on the lookout for invaders, such as bacteria and viruses. Once the immune system recognizes that there is an invader, it attacks it.

One of the main characters in the immune system is the white blood cells. The white blood cells are also known as leukocytes. They protect the body against disease and illness. The white blood cells flow through the bloodstream to fight bacteria, viruses, and other invaders that are a threat to our health. The white blood cells are made in the bone marrow and they are stored in the blood and the lymph tissues. The bone marrow is constantly making new white blood cells because some of them can exist only a day, or sometimes just a couple of hours. When the body is in distress and a certain area is under attack, white blood cells rush through the bloodstream and help destroy whatever harmful substance has attacked the body. With this action, the white blood cells are preventing illness.

There are many types of white blood cells. They are all made to protect the body against invaders. For example, the lymphocytes create antibodies to fight against viruses, bacteria, and some other harmful invaders that can potentially attack the body. Another example is the neutrophils, they kill and digest fungi and bacteria. They represent the first line of defense when an invader or any kind of infection strikes. They are the most widespread and numerous types of white blood cells.

Monocytes help to break down any bacteria and they usually have a much longer lifespan than other white blood cells.

The white blood cells that attack and kill parasites and cancer cells are called eosinophils. They also help the body with allergic responses.

Last but not least is basophils. Basophils are small cells that alarm the body when an infectious agent invade and attack the blood. This type of white blood cells chemicals like histamine. These kinds of chemicals help the body control the immune response.

A problem can occur if the number of white blood cells is low. And this could happen for various reasons. For example, something may destroy the cells more quickly than the body can replenish them. Sometimes, the bone marrow is not able to make enough white blood cells and that is unhealthy for the body. When this happens, the person who has a low level of white blood cells is at great risk for any kind of illness or disease. This can be a very serious threat to the general well-being.

In addition to this, many people diagnosed with Ulcerative Colitis have a weak and abnormal immune system. The immune system in someone diagnosed with Ulcerative Colitis is not functioning as it should and this is a very serious problem. Because the purpose of the immune system is to defend the body against invaders and toxic materials, without it the body is just open for any kind of attack. What happens is that the immune system attacks the healthy tissues, the ones that are supposed to protect us. This is a mistake that can occur with the Ulcerative Colitis condition. Normally, the immune system fights off the invaders by realizing white blood cells into the blood. In that way, the white blood cells can protect the body and destroy the cause of infection. However, Ulcerative Colitis is weakening the immune system. The immune system mistakes the so-called friendly bacteria with invaders. This causes inflammation in the inner lining of the colon.

The immune system has the purpose of defending the body from infections and disease and all the things that do not belong in the body. But instead of that, it attacks itself. The white blood cells actually attack the intestinal lining and that leads to ongoing inflammation.

Some kind of infection triggers the immune system and for some reason, it does not turn off. This causes colon inflammation which is the main symptom of Ulcerative Colitis.

Moreover, a virus or a germ that could be found in the environment can also attack the body. And because it cannot protect itself, the body can get affected and this can also raise the chances of getting the Ulcerative Colitis condition. The immune systems of many persons with ulcerative colitis are dysfunctional. Experts aren't sure if immunological disorders are to blame for the sickness. They're also unsure if ulcerative colitis can lead to immune system disorders. The immune system reacts improperly to chemical signals, resulting in gastrointestinal inflammation. There appears to be a genetic component as well, for someone with a family history of Ulcerative Colitis being more likely to experience this abnormal immune response.

A weaker immune system can be caused by a variety of factors such as medication, recent surgery, age, genetics, or a chronic illness. An illness like Ulcerative Colitis can cause significant immune system difficulties and have many negative impacts on a person's health. It's unclear why all of this is possible, yet it is. And because this is a long-term condition and the causes of it are still not very clear, there is not much that can be done. Many microorganisms in the stomach are completely safe and harmless. But in inflammatory bowel disease such as Ulcerative Colitis, the immune system targets the bacteria, that are not dangerous, inside the colon. And instead of letting it help to body, the immune system attacks the tissues of the colon. And this causes the colon to become inflamed.

When the immune system detects a virus or illness, it goes into overdrive and fights it. An immunological reaction is what this is referred to as. This reaction can sometimes encompass healthy cells and tissues, resulting in autoimmune disease.

When your body's natural defense system can't distinguish the difference between your own cells and foreign cells, it attacks normal cells, creating autoimmune disease. It is believed that Ulcerative Colitis is an autoimmune disease. Although the cause is still not clear, because Ulcerative Colitis causes the immune system to attacks its own harmless bacteria, the experts have a reason to believe that this might actually be an autoimmune disease. Ulcerative colitis is an autoimmune disease that is likely to cause the immune system to assault healthy gut tissue. The large intestine becomes inflamed, resulting in the symptoms of Ulcerative Colitis. This condition can weaken the immune system if not treated properly. Certain Ulcerative Colitis medicines have been shown to suppress the immune system. But, there is not a solution that is beneficial to cure the whole disease. Although ulcerative colitis is hardly ever fatal, it is a severe condition that can lead to life-threatening consequences. When our immune system reacts to something that isn't infectious, it might unintentionally create illness symptoms. This sort of immunological response is linked to allergic responses. Similarly, our immune systems can occasionally overreact, overloading our bodies and leading to death. Autoimmune disorders, inflammatory diseases, and cancer can all be caused by immune system problems. Immunodeficiency is a condition in which the immune system is not as effective as it should be, resulting in frequent and sometimes fatal infections. This can be extreme and harmful to a person's health. Especially if you have been diagnosed with a disease like Ulcerative Colitis. Because this condition already has a wide range of symptoms, both mild and severe, and because it is a long-term illness. An autoimmune reaction can impair organ function or cause irregular organ development in addition to damaging body tissue. Blood arteries, connective tissue, joints, muscles, red blood cells, skin, and the thyroid gland are all often impacted by autoimmune diseases, like Ulcerative Colitis.

Living a healthy lifestyle and eating a balanced and healthy diet, exercising regularly, reducing stress, and getting plenty of rest can help treat the symptoms. Using medications such as pain relievers and anti-inflammatory drugs can relieve the severe abdominal pain an autoimmune disease, like Ulcerative Colitis can cause. Some people who are diagnosed with this condition find therapy a lot helpful. Blood transfusions may be required in situations when the blood is affected. Ulcerative colitis cannot be prevented, therefore patients should see their doctor frequently to establish a treatment plan to assist control the disease's symptoms and consequences.

In most cases, diseases cannot be prevented, especially not autoimmune ones. Because there is not a known clue what causes it and why. But, you can always try to do something that will make you feel better. You can take care of your mental health as well, because that is really important, particularly when you are dealing with some kind of disease. Because of the fact that Ulcerative Colitis is unpredictable, you can never know for sure when the symptoms will show. Some patients can get into remission when their symptoms go away completely. Days, weeks, months, or even years might pass in this manner. Remission, on the other hand, isn't necessarily permanent. Many patients have flare-ups from time to time, which means their UC symptoms reappear. Flare-ups come in a variety of lengths. Flare-ups can also vary in severity from individual to person.

Although symptoms might appear at any time, there is a way to extend the duration between flare-ups. Knowing how to manage the return of the symptoms and recognizing factors that might provoke a flare-up are key to getting a handle on Ulcerative Colitis. Learning how to deal with Ulcerative Colitis flare-ups can improve your mood and quality of life.

Keeping a food journal might help you identify the items that can cause flare-ups. Knowing that Ulcerative Colitis makes most of the symptoms to be triggered by food, can actually help you manage the unwanted symptoms. Because of the fact that Ulcerative Colitis is a lifelong autoimmune disease, it is necessary to take care of your health. And for that matter, you should learn how to control all the things that you can, including the intake of food and beverages that may cause a symptom.

2.2 The impact Ulcerative Colitis has on your general health

Ulcerative Colitis symptoms usually tend to be mild but, for some people, the symptoms can be very severe. And despite that, Ulcerative Colitis is a lifelong condition, so it can have a huge effect on a person's general health. It is not easy to live with a chronic disease, such as Ulcerative Colitis because it is very unpredictable. And for that matter, you should be very careful.

You may need to adjust your Ulcerative Colitis diet if you have additional health issues or dietary sensitivities that necessitate careful attention to what you eat.

Although stress does not cause Ulcerative Colitis, being stressed while having this disease can be a problem. Learning how to successfully manage stress levels may reduce the frequency of Ulcerative Colitis symptoms. You can reduce stress by exercising regularly and also, exercising is a great mood booster. Even 10 or 15 minutes of exercising can help you relieve stress and it might reduce the symptoms. In addition to this, you should practice some relaxation techniques, such as yoga or meditation. This can help you be less stressed and more relaxed. Yoga and meditation can provide you better mental health and more positive energy. Taking care of your mental health is really important because it all comes down to how you feel. Even though Ulcerative Colitis is an unpredictable disease, you should not overthink it. Living with Ulcerative Colitis can be really frustrating and isolating and it can increase the level of anxiety. Communication with someone with the same condition or a similar one can help you feel better. It always helps to know that you are not alone. People with the same condition can understand more easily what you are going through. And it can also help reduce the level of anxiety. Anxiety can occur because you cannot be able to know when and how exactly a symptom might be triggered.

Ulcerative Colitis is a long-term, chronic disease for which there is no treatment. The majority of persons with Ulcerative Colitis have symptoms that come and go throughout their lives. The unpredictability of this condition can have a major impact on one's quality of life. It may feel as if you are being kept captive by your own body, depending on the intensity of your symptoms. As a result of this situation, some persons with UC may experience anxiety and depression. Living with a long-term disease like Ulcerative Colitis, which is uncertain and possibly devastating, maybe emotionally draining.

Anxiety and depression are more common in people with Ulcerative Colitis than in the general population. One-third of patients with inflammatory bowel disease, such as Ulcerative Colitis, have anxiety symptoms, while a quarter has depressive symptoms. Concerns about the emergence and severity of Ulcerative Colitis symptoms can create anxiety and stress, and studies suggest that anxiety and stress can cause inflammatory bowel disorders like Ulcerative Colitis to flare up.

Some people feel overwhelmed by this disease and happen to have a poor self-image. More are likely to be in denial about the effects that Ulcerative Colitis can bring on their mental health and that can lead to dependent personality disorder or DPD. These people often feel incapable of taking care of themselves and they feel submissive. They might have trouble making a simple decision and depend on someone else for very basic and not so important things. They also tend to feel helpless most of the time. It is important and necessary to get treatments for the effects on your mental health that are caused by the Ulcerative Colitis condition. Receiving help for this condition can help the dependent person with Ulcerative Colitis be more self-reliant and boost self-confidence.

Anxiety and stress brought on by Ulcerative Colitis can sometimes lead to depression. Feeling unhappy, hopeless, and no longer enjoying activities you used to like are all signs of depression. If you are feeling depressed, you should probably talk to a professional. Or if you are not really comfortable talking to a professional, you can always contact someone that is also affected by Ulcerative Colitis. There are also support groups that can help your depression and make you feel better.

Infertility can also be a possible problem that can occur with Ulcerative Colitis. It is not caused by it, but it can play some role. The possibility of a woman with Ulcerative Colitis becoming pregnant is typically unaffected by the disease. However, infertility can be a side effect of surgery carried out to create an ilea-anal pouch. If you have surgery to reroute your small intestine through a hole in your stomach, this risk is greatly reduced.

There may be times when you need to make major, but only temporary, dietary adjustments. For instance, suppose you got pregnant. Irritable bowel disease symptoms may worsen at this period, in part because of hormonal fluctuations that may damage the stomach. However, you may experience fewer flares during this period — everyone is different.

There are a few coping practices that can help you improve your mental health and learn how to avoid triggering Ulcerative Colitis symptoms. To help people cope with Ulcerative Colitis and improve their mental health eating healthy and avoiding food that can cause and trigger a symptom seems to be the most useful method. Minimizing alcohol and caffeine consumption is also good prevention from unwanted symptom triggers. Into the bargain, you should get as much sleep as possible every night. Another thing that can help you is using supplements, but this is only a solution if your health professional recommends it.

Some signs of mental health problems can include extreme fatigue and you also might have difficulty concentrating. Persistent sadness and feeling of worthlessness and guilt can also be signs that your mental health might require a need of professional help. Ulcerative Colitis diagnosed person can also lose interest in things and activities that used to find fun and amusing once.

Drugs and alcohol abuse can be a sign of a mental health problem, as well. And this can be very dangerous and can lead to serious problems because drugs and alcohol are able to trigger Ulcerative Colitis symptoms and cause unwanted flare-ups. In addition to this, some people tend to isolate themselves and lose contact with friends and family. This can affect someone's mental health and can lead to something more serious, like suicidal thoughts. For preventing this, you should communicate with support groups and healthcare professionals, but your family and friends as well.

Physical symptoms such as headaches and backaches might be caused by mental health issues. It does not necessarily mean that you have a mental health disorder if you occasionally encounter one or more of these symptoms. If you happen to suffer from several of the previously mentioned symptoms for an extended length of time, or if you have suicidal thoughts, you should seek medical advice. The first step to getting assistance for anxiety or depression caused by Ulcerative Colitis is to speak with your doctor. Adjusting your medicine to help manage inflammation may be part of the treatment. To boost your mood, your doctor may prescribe an antidepressant or anti-anxiety medicine.

Doctors may also suggest seeing a mental health expert for treatment. These sessions might teach you coping techniques and ways to cope with stressful situations. You will also discover how to improve your mental patterns and eliminate negative ideas that deepen sadness. Home remedies, diet changes, and improving your lifestyle, in addition to the usual therapy, may help you improve your mental health.

Accepting that you are not able to control every single thing can help you reduce anxiety. In addition to this, you should learn how to challenge negative thoughts as they arise, because you are not able to predict some things, just like the Ulcerative Colitis condition and you should just celebrate your best efforts. Learning about triggers and how you can manage them is yet another thing that you can do to better your mental health and be more relaxed. Being able to avoid some of the triggers might help you enjoy your life a little more. You might have mental health benefits from making time for fun activities and things you want to do every day. Or maybe by helping someone else that is dealing with Ulcerative Colitis, you can also help yourself.

Chapter 3: Relieve the symptoms by eating better

3.1 Which diet aggravates the symptoms? -Food to avoid

If you have Ulcerative Colitis, you may be able to control your illness by avoiding specific foods that can help minimize the risk of flare-ups and inflammation. Food does not cause this disease, but if you have Ulcerative Colitis, it will be worth your while to pay attention to what you consume. Some food can actually help you and set off the flares. You have to watch out for items that can be troublemakers if you have this disease. Some foods can really be bad for Ulcerative Colitis patients. Ulcerative Colitis is not caused by any particular food or diet, but the symptoms will be affected by what you usually eat and drink. It will be better for your general health if you try to avoid the items that will trigger the symptoms and cause flare-ups.

Mostly they are the thing that does not go well with any disease, like alcohol. Drinking alcohol can higher up the risks and lower the chance of treating the disease with medication. Different kinds of alcohol may have different effects on you, but they may all stimulate your gut and cause diarrhea. However, you may be able to consume little quantities in moderation.

Caffeine is also a bad choice if you have Ulcerative Colitis. Even if you do not take caffeine in big doses is not good for your mind and your body. Caffeine is found in tea, chocolate, and energy drinks, not just in coffee. Caffeine is a stimulant and for someone who has this disease it will speed up the transit time in the colon. Tea and other caffeinated beverages, as well as goods containing guarana, a stimulant commonly found in energy drinks, fall under this category.

Dairy products have always been a tricky food. Even if you are not lactose intolerant, dairy can cause skin troubles. Dairy might be a symptom trigger for you, so if you suspect that you should remove all types of dairy, including milk, yogurt, cheese, and butter. Most people believe that if they have Ulcerative Colitis, they are always lactose intolerant, but this is not the case. Lactose intolerance is caused by a lack of a certain enzyme. And the only way to find out is to conduct an experiment in which you drink a glass of milk and then observe how you feel afterward. If you feel worse, it is better to avoid dairy.

Dried peas, beans, and lentils are high-fiber and high-protein foods. You wouldn't be able to digest the sugars in beans and they can cause gas. They're not an ideal food for someone having an Ulcerative Colitis flare. But they're still an important staple in many diets, especially for vegetarians and vegans.

Meat is a bad food choice. Especially fatty meats. They can trigger most of the symptoms. The fat from the meat can't be properly absorbed during a flare and this can only make the symptoms worse. Red meat is also bad because it is high in sulfate and that can trigger gas.

Also, you should avoid whole-grain foods, such as brown rice, buckwheat, oats, quinoa, and wild rice. These foods can irritate more the disease and may trigger a flare-up. You should avoid plain barley, millet, wheat berries, and spelt.

The fiber in nuts is very hard to digest, so in that matter, you should avoid walnuts, pecans, pistachios, macadamia nuts, hazelnuts, almonds, cashews, and peanuts. Just like nuts, seeds can also aggravate symptoms. They can cause bloating, gas and diarrhea. Some of the seeds you have to avoid are millet, sunflower seeds, sesame seeds, pumpkin seeds, and flax seeds. Nuts and seeds are high in unsaturated fats, fiber, and protein, all of which are beneficial to your health. However, because of their high fiber content, they might irritate the digestive system. Nuts must be chewed thoroughly or blended into fine bits for most patients with Ulcerative Colitis, and you may need to avoid them entirely during a flare.

Avoid eating entire seeds if you have a flare-up of Ulcerative Colitis. Even avoiding the small fruit seeds in the fruit itself, as well as in smoothies, jams, and yogurts prepared with fresh fruit will benefit. Seeds, on the other hand, are usually not an issue if ground finely enough. Some people have never experienced a bad reaction to ground flaxseed or tahini, which is prepared from sesame seeds.

Avoid foods that are difficult to digest, such as corn, mushrooms, roughage such as broccoli and cabbage, and tiny, hard foods such as seeds and nuts. Their high fiber content can make them really difficult for digestion and can cause abdominal pain.

Although sulfate is a required nutrient in a human diet, it can also feed a certain kind of bacteria that create H2S toxic gas in the person that is diagnosed with Ulcerative Colitis.

Mayonnaise and Alfredo sauce, for example, are high-fat condiments and sauces that might aggravate Ulcerative Colitis symptoms. Some people have issues with peanut butter, which is high in healthy fats as well.

Another food intolerance for those who have digestive symptoms is gluten. And it is becoming more common. Gluten is a protein found in many kinds of food. It is also added to already prepared products like sauces, soups, condiments, and proteins. Gluten can be a symptom trigger, so for that matter, you have to remove everything gluten-containing grains. Such as cereals and baked goods.

Most fruits contain a lot of fiber. Although they are healthy for you, some fruits belong on the list of foods you should avoid if you have Ulcerative Colitis. For example, you have to avoid raw and dried fruit and also, fruit that has seeds that can't be removed, like most berries. Citrus fruits are difficult to digest as well. They might induce stomach discomfort in some people due to their high fiber content. If your stomach is upset, avoid oranges, grapefruit, and other citrus fruits.

Fibrous vegetables are also not a good idea for people diagnosed with Ulcerative Colitis. They are also full of fiber and hard to digest. You should avoid all undercooked or raw vegetables, including corn. Another "stringy" vegetable that might be difficult to stomach is onions. It can be a very big problem digesting an onion.

Another thing that can irritate the digestive tract is carbonation. Beverages such as sodas and beers contain carbonation. They contain sugar and caffeine or some kind of artificial sweeteners. Most of these cause gas. Not only do most include caffeine, sugar, or artificial sweeteners, which can produce gas and bloating, but the bubbles can also cause cramping and bloating. If you're going to drink soda, keep it to a minimum and avoid using a straw, which might cause extra air bubbles to enter your stomach.

Another high fiber is popcorn. Popcorn can't be digested properly and it can cause bowel movement urgency and diarrhea. Your digestive system may have difficulties adapting if you start consuming a lot of them. The end effect is bloating and gas. And in addition to this, you should lower the intake of fiber.

Chocolate is also bad for someone who has Ulcerative Colitis. It contains caffeine and sugar. Both of these can irritate the digestive tract and cause cramping. More often, it can also cause more bowel movements.

Refined sugar can also cause diarrhea. You could experience cramps and diarrhea if you eat too much sugar-free gum produced with sorbitol. Food containing this artificial sweetener has the potential to produce the same issues.

Peppermint can relax the muscle at the top of the stomach, allowing food to pass back into the esophagus. This can result in heartburn. Chocolate and coffee are two more causes. If you lose weight, eat smaller quantities, and don't lay down after eating, experts suggest you can reduce the pressure that pulls the food back up.

Another kind of food that is bad for those diagnosed with this disease is spicy food. Any kind of spicy foods, pepper, and hot sauces. These can cause diarrhea and worse symptoms. After eating spicy food, some people get indigestion or heartburn, especially if they eat a large meal. Capsaicin, a fiery common ingredient in chili peppers, has been linked to cancer in studies.

Fried meals are extremely difficult to digest. They contain a lot of fat and might cause diarrhea. Sauces with a lot of fat, fatty types of meat, and buttery or creamy desserts can all be problematic.

People's eating choices appear to have an influence on when symptoms flare up. Diets will vary quite a bit since not everyone reacts to food in the same manner. What triggers symptoms in one individual may be different from what triggers symptoms in another. It's all dependent on a variety of things: Because a person with Ulcerative Colitis may also be suffering from another illness. And these kinds of scenarios are more difficult. Dairy seems like it can be a symptom trigger in most e cases and especially if you are lactose intolerant, your chances of experiencing severe symptoms are increased, therefore you should avoid dairy at all costs. However, there are some people whose symptoms do not get triggered by eating dairy and they are also affected by Ulcerative Colitis. It is not clear why things like these can happen. Every person is different and so is their reaction to different types of food.

There is no one particular diet that is the best choice for those with Ulcerative Colitis, but identifying and avoiding the items that can trigger symptoms can help alleviate pain. Doctors are not sure what causes this condition, but they believe it has something to do with the environment, westernized foods and lifestyles, and heredity. A healthy diet can contribute to the treatment of Ulcerative Colitis. There are many, many kinds of foods that you are not allowed to eat if you are diagnosed with Ulcerative Colitis, because triggering symptoms can be bad and can make more serious problems. Not just to the colon or rectum, but for the rest of the organs. It can be very dangerous and it can make your health worse.

Ulcerative Colitis can cause many bad symptoms triggered by food. You can still enjoy many different foods and you can choose a diet that is perfect for your health and that will not cause further problems. You have to be very careful when it comes to choosing a particular diet, because of the fact that Ulcerative Colitis symptoms can be easily triggered. And also, if you are diagnosed with another disease as well, you have to be careful about that and the things that can cause a bad affection for it. It is not easy to live with this kind of disease, alluding to the point that Ulcerative Colitis is a chronic illness. It is important to make it easier for yourself to live with it. And for that matter, you have to have a balanced diet plan. Which is a good thing. You can plan what you eat and how many nutrients you consume. It does not all have to be that bad. In that order, read the next chapter to find out more about the food that can be good for a person that is diagnosed with Ulcerative Colitis condition.

3.2 What To Eat? – Beneficial Nutrition Habits To Get On The Right Path

It might be difficult to determine which meals would best feed your body, especially if you have Ulcerative Colitis. Living with an inflammatory bowel disease, like Ulcerative Colitis may necessitate dietary adjustments. To alleviate your symptoms, you may need to avoid specific meals or take extra precautions to ensure that you are obtaining enough nutrients. As previously said, no one diet is suitable for everyone who is impacted by this condition. With inflammatory bowel disease, food and nutrition are extremely important, but there is not a specific diet that works for every Ulcerative Colitis diagnosed person. As said before, most foods can trigger symptoms and make Ulcerative Colitis even worse. However, there are many foods that you actually can consume and not trigger the disease. Some changes in your diet can help you control the condition. Not only can nutrition have an impact on inflammatory bowel disease symptoms, but it also has an impact on your general health and well-being. The symptoms of Ulcerative Colitis can lead to significant problems if you do not have enough nutrients, such as nutritional deficiency, weight loss, and malnutrition. Although a specific diet is not considered to play a role in the development of Ulcerative Colitis, several lifestyle interventions can benefit in its management.

Food that contains nutrients provides us energy and aid in the growth and repair of our bodies. A healthy, well-balanced diet ensures that we obtain all of the nutrients our bodies require. Depending on how active your Ulcerative Colitis is, your diet may change. You may not be able to consume a balanced diet during a flare-up. It is important to take care of your health as much as you can. Taking better care of our bodies implies more energy and a greater ability to achieve our everyday goals. It implies that we will be able to focus better on any specific assignment and that our duties will be completed in less time. Healthy living should be a part of your daily routine. A healthy lifestyle can help you avoid some diseases. And for those you cannot avoid, such as Ulcerative Colitis, it is better for you and your health if you are more responsible and careful about the things you consume.

Here is some dietary advice for you that you might find useful.

Food is an excellent kind of medicine. When you have Ulcerative Colitis, this is especially relevant. Symptoms of Ulcerative Colitis, such as diarrhea and vomiting, might cause you to lose nutrients. As a result, it is necessary to eat enough food. Vegetables, in particular, provide some of the most beneficial nutrients and micronutrients.

For example, you should drink plenty of fluids since you lose lots of them through diarrhea. It is really easy to become dehydrated if you have Ulcerative Colitis. Normally, water is always the best source of fluids. When you have Ulcerative Colitis, it is essential to consume enough water. Drinking plenty of water will help you replace the fluids you have lost due to diarrhea. It is possible that water alone will not be enough. When you have diarrhea, your body loses electrolytes including salt, potassium, and magnesium.

Staying hydrated may be as simple as drinking water with electrolytes. At your local pharmacy, you can get that mixture in the form of an oral rehydration drink. Electrolytes and fluid are also included in sports beverages such as Gatorade and Powerade. Everyone's hydration requirements vary, so aim for eight 8-ounce glasses of water each day. When your urine is light yellow in color, you know you are well hydrated. When you know that you will lose additional fluids from sweating or if your diarrhea is flaring up, it's incredibly important to drink plenty of water. When it is hot outside or you are exercising, bring a water bottle with you and drink regularly. For those with digestive problems, carbonated drinks, caffeine, and alcoholic beverages might be unpleasant. While it is vital to keep hydrated, limit yourself to water or liquids suggested by your doctor, such as electrolyte replacement drinks and liquid nutritional supplements. It is important to remember that drinking water is not the only process of keeping your body hydrated. Add additional fluid sources, such as fruit juice, clear broth, ice pops, and low-fiber fruits like melon, when you are bored with the taste of water. Although you should make water your preferred beverage. Water infused with natural ingredients like ginger, turmeric, lemon, and other citrus fruits is delicious and highly purifying for your intestines.

Even if you are in remission and your symptoms have reduced or vanished, it is necessary to maintain a balanced and nutrient-rich diet. Slowly introduce new meals. Remember to drink plenty of water, broth, tomato juice, and rehydration products to remain hydrated.

Fiber-rich meals can assist you in staying healthy and hydrated. Oat bran, beans, barley, almonds, and whole grains are examples of healthy foods. Unless you have an ostomy, intestinal constriction, or your doctor recommends a low-fiber diet due to strictures or recent surgery. Fiber may help prolong periods of Ulcerative Colitis remission and provide additional advantages, according to some studies. Insoluble fiber, on the other hand, might worsen Ulcerative Colitis symptoms during a flare. Before making any changes to your fiber intake, consult with a doctor or a nutritionist. Fiber has several health advantages, including lowering blood pressure, lowering cholesterol, increasing insulin sensitivity, assisting those with obesity in losing weight, and boosting immunological function.

When you are experiencing symptoms, go for low-fiber bread, spaghetti, and other carbs. This usually indicates they are produced with processed white flour rather than entire grains. Another low-fiber choice that might be calming and simple to digest is white rice. Brown rice, wild rice, and rice pilaf should be avoided. For toast, go with sourdough rather than a fiber-rich choice like multigrain. Low-sugar cereals, grits, and oatmeal sachets may also be suitable. Any cereal, bread, or granola that contains dried fruit or nuts should be avoided.

Omega-3 fatty acids found in salmon and albacore tuna can help decrease inflammation during a flare and may even help you stay in remission. Mackerel, herring, sardines, flaxseed oil, powdered flaxseed, and walnuts are all good sources of omega-3s. During a flare, some people may be unable to eat whole nuts or flaxseeds, although they may be acceptable if ground up. Aim to eat salmon once or twice a week, and if your budget permits, go for wild salmon over farmed salmon.

Because proteins are commonly lost during flares of Ulcerative Colitis, lean meats and poultry are advised. Increasing your protein intake can aid in the recovery of nutrients lost during a flare. When you have symptoms as well as when you are symptom-free, lean protein like skinless chicken breast merely cooked can help. Avoid overcooking the meat, frying it, and adding butter, spices, or heavy sauces to it. Vegetarians and vegans can use soy-based protein instead of animal protein. Legumes and whole grains are also good sources of non-animal proteins. Keep in mind that if you do not consume meat and instead rely on plant-based protein staples like beans and lentils, these meals might induce flatulence. Other non-meat protein alternatives include tofu or tempeh, which are frequently soft or "silken," making them readily digestible and flexible.

Eggs are another good source of protein, and they're usually tolerated well even during flare-ups. Some eggs have omega-3 fatty acids added to them, which can help decrease inflammation.

Probiotics are beneficial bacteria that can help with digestion and can be found in yogurt, kefir, sauerkraut, and miso. Sugar can worsen Ulcerative Colitis symptoms, so look for yogurts with less added sugars.

Unsweetened applesauce is tasteless and may be ingested after an Ulcerative Colitis flare-up, however, it may be difficult to handle during a flare-up for some people. During a flare, your gastrointestinal tract is likely to be irritated, so soft, readily digested meals like applesauce are a good choice. However, make sure to get one that isn't sweetened, as sugar might exacerbate inflammation. You may also create your own sugar-free applesauce by pureeing peeled, sliced apples with little water.

Instant oatmeal comprises refined grains and, since it contains less fiber, is frequently easier to prepare than steel-cut or old-fashioned oatmeal.

Squash is a nutritious food that is typically easily tolerated by Ulcerative Colitis patients. It has a high amount of fiber, vitamin C, and beta carotene. Cooked butternut, zucchini, spaghetti, acorn, winter, and summer squashes are the most tolerable. During an Ulcerative Colitis flare, raw squash may exacerbate symptoms.

Some people may handle juice and smoothies during a flare, and they can help you maintain a healthy diet. Carrot juice is high in vitamin A and antioxidants, and it is well tolerated by many patients with Ulcerative Colitis.

Coconut Oil Chocolate Candies is a wonderful dessert choice. Commercial chocolate, which is loaded with refined cane sugar, can be difficult to consume for many individuals with Ulcerative Colitis, but there are still methods to enjoy chocolate using cocoa powder and raw honey, as long as the honey does not provoke symptoms. This recipe makes tiny, melt-in-your-mouth chocolates with raw honey as a sweetener. The recipe for this dessert is just a couple pages away. Bananas, melons, blueberries, strawberries, oranges, and grapes are some of the fruits accessible. While fulfilling your sweet craving, these fruits contain vitamins and antioxidants. Furthermore, unlike fruits with higher sugar content, they do not cause gas, which is an Ulcerative Colitis trigger.

Flare-ups of inflammatory bowel disease can lead to malnutrition, so it is crucial to eat nutrient-dense meals even while you're in remission. Eating a rainbow of colors can help you receive a wide range of vitamins and minerals.

Biophenols are found in the fruits and leaves of olive trees, and they are the most abundant source of antioxidants in the human diet from fruits and vegetables.

Curcumin, a component of turmeric, is another anti-inflammatory that has been promoted for a variety of illnesses. Some small trials have indicated that it can assist people with Ulcerative Colitis go into and stay in remission. Turmeric may be simply added to cooked vegetables, scrambled eggs, smoothies, tea, and other dishes.

While you should avoid lactose in other dairy products, certain studies have indicated that the active culture Lactobacillus GG present in some yogurts can help your gut's microbiota rebalance. This permits the beneficial bacteria in your stomach to break down your meal without making you feel bloated.

Kimchi and sauerkraut are good sources of probiotics, which aid digestion and nutrient absorption while also supporting gut health. Both of these ingredients are simple to put into scrambled eggs or tacos.

Prebiotic foods like raw Jerusalem artichokes, leeks, dandelion root, and onions can be used to test the waters if you are not close to experiencing a flare-up. These meals are difficult to digest, yet they nourish the beneficial bacteria in your stomach, promoting microbiome balance. However, if you are following a low-FODMAP diet, these items are not the best options.

Thousands of patients with bowel illness and other diseases have greatly improved their quality of life by following a particular carbohydrate diet. Many people believe they have been cured. It's a diet designed to help people with Ulcerative Colitis. It is, however, a highly nutritious, balanced, and safe diet that helps everyone's health. The chemical nature of the meals determines which foods are allowed on the particular carbohydrate diet. The molecular structure of carbohydrates is used to classify them. Some foods you can eat while you are practicing this diet are nuts and nut flours, milk, and other dairy products that are low in sugar lactose, meat, eggs, butter, oil, and most fruits and vegetables.

Consider adopting a Mediterranean diet if you want to try something new. It is low in triggering saturated fats and high in vegetables, lean proteins, and good fats that may reduce inflammation. The Mediterranean diet is proven to bring down inflammation in general. Fruits, vegetables, legumes, nuts and seeds, whole grains, fish, poultry, dairy products, eggs, olive oil, and other beneficial fats.

Nut-based butter like peanut butter, almond butter, cashew butter, and others are high in protein and healthy fats. To avoid having to digest tough nut bits during a flare, go for smooth peanut butter rather than chunky peanut butter. Wrap peanut butter in a tortilla or eat it on toast. Nut butter on low-fiber crackers, such as saltines, is another acceptable option.

If you cannot stomach most foods during an Ulcerative Colitis flare, bland foods like boiled white rice are a good alternative. If you want to add some taste, sprinkle it with turmeric, a yellow spice whose main component, curcumin, has been found to help in Ulcerative Colitis therapy. Curcumin combined with an anti-inflammatory was shown to be more effective than using an anti-inflammatory alone in treating Ulcerative Colitis, according to experts. In India, where the frequency of inflammatory bowel disease is lower than in the United States or Europe, turmeric is extensively utilized.

Although most dietitians advise against eating raw fruits during a flare, very ripe, mushy bananas are typically tolerated. Bananas are also high in carbs, which give energy together with protein and lipids. Soft fruits, such as canned pears or peaches, may not irritate you.

Carrots and spinach, for example, are soft, cooked vegetables that may give vital nutrients like vitamins A and K. Just make sure the veggies are fully cooked — until they can be mashed with a fork — to break down any potentially irritating fiber.

If you are practicing a gluten-free diet you can consume fruits and vegetables, some beans, seeds, and legumes. As well as, eggs, fish, poultry, and meat. You can also eat most low-fat dairy products or non-dairy. And also, you can eat grains such as quinoa, corn, buckwheat, flax, and amaranth.

There is a chance that some kind of food can help you avoid flare-ups. Some healthy foods may have anti-inflammatory properties that can aid in the management of Ulcerative Colitis' underlying inflammation. Unprocessed foods make up a large portion of this list. They also have a lot of color in them. The pigments that give fruits and vegetables their color have anti-inflammatory and other health-promoting properties. This type of eating promotes anti-inflammatory pathways in our bodies, which can be beneficial when dealing with inflammatory bowel diseases, such as Ulcerative Colitis.

Antioxidant and anti-inflammatory compounds may be found in abundance in vegetables and fruits. Beta-carotene, anthocyanin, and other chemicals found in dark leafy greens and cruciferous vegetables, such as broccoli, cabbage, Brussel sprouts, cauliflower, carrots, beets, berries, onions, peas, squashes, sea vegetables, and salad greens prevent illness at the molecular level. If your stomach has trouble digesting fruits and vegetables, try eating them in tiny amounts. Cooking veggies also makes them more digestible. Although cruciferous veggies produce gas and stink, many people can tolerate tiny doses of them.

Beans and legumes are also high in folic acid, magnesium, potassium, and soluble fiber, all of which aid in stool formation and softening. Beans, such as black, white, kidney, adzuki, chickpeas, black-eyed peas, and lentils, contain a wide range of nutrients.

Because whole grains, as opposed to those that have been coarsely crushed into flour, are absorbed slowly, they assist to maintain blood sugar and energy levels. Whole grains include barley, brown rice, buckwheat, quinoa, millet, and steel-cut oats, to name a few.

Fresh herbs and spices give flavor to your cuisine without the need for salt. Tumeric and ginger also have the added benefit of being anti-inflammatory. They're also chock-full of antioxidants. Antioxidants can also be found in basil, chili peppers, curry powder, rosemary, and thyme.

Fat is an essential part of a good and balanced diet. Extra virgin olive oil is ideal for sautéing over low heat and creating cold dressings or sauces since it is the least processed and has a beautiful, robust taste. Coconut oil is worth a try, particularly if you have trouble digesting fat. It digests more readily and thoroughly without the need for bile salts than other plant oils since it is a medium-chain triglyceride. As a result, it may be beneficial to those suffering from malnutrition or malabsorption. Because coconut is solid at room temperature, it is versatile and may be used in place of butter in both sautéing and baking.

As mentioned previously, omega-3 fats are essential since our bodies cannot produce them. Nuts, avocados, freshly ground flaxseed, and seafood all contain them. Because of their low heavy metal level, wild salmon and sardines are preferred as omega-3 sources over other fish. They can help you avoid unwanted flare-ups. However, you should not take any artificial fats. Artificial trans fats should be avoided at all costs, as they raise the risk of heart disease. Trans fat is utilized to increase the shelf life of crackers, cookies, and other processed foods.

Fermented foods are high in helpful microorganisms that flourish in our gastrointestinal system. Eating fermented foods repopulates the digestive system with these microorganisms, ensuring that the gut bacteria population is balanced. Fermented foods have long been a part of most civilizations' diets. Italians consume antipasto. Japanese consume miso, tempeh, and natto. Eastern Europeans consume kefir (or kephir) or yogurt; Koreans consume kimchee. On the other side, Germans consume sauerkraut.

Vegetarians and vegans who are affected by Ulcerative Colitis disease should pay more attention to what they can and cannot consume. Because some of the foods they usually consume in exchange for animal protein can cause flare-ups and can trigger a symptom. Iron is needed to fight anemia, which can occur as a result of nutritional loss during a flare. Spinach, artichokes, raisins, and kale are among iron-rich plant-based meals that are simpler to digest than beans. Cashews, potatoes, and quinoa are other wonderful choices.

Fat is necessary for nutritional absorption, but eating too much at each meal might result in frequent visits to the bathroom. Try to limit yourself to no more than a couple teaspoons at a time, or find a level that suits you. Hemp seeds and coconut flesh are two exceptions, as they are both easily digestible fats that contain high-quality nutrients.

Many patients with Ulcerative Colitis are unable to eat entire meals at first, therefore meal replacement smoothies and protein drinks are prescribed to help them obtain their nutrition and avoid dehydration. Dehydration can cause tiredness and nutritional loss, so drink plenty of water and eat nutrient-dense smoothies. Plant-based protein powders (pea and hemp are often simple to digest) may be less difficult to digest than whey, sprouted grains, or sprouted bean-based protein powders. Vegetable broth can also assist offer nutrients that you might be missing out on since you couldn't eat entire meals at first.

For those with Ulcerative Colitis, a plant-based diet might be difficult because a low residue diet is typically suggested. Because most plant-based foods are high in fiber, finding a happy amount of fiber that keeps you healthy without provoking a flare can be difficult. Peel all fruits and vegetables before eating them, cook vegetables before eating them, eat more soup, and replace wheat, bran cereals, steel-cut oats, and whole quinoa seeds with lower-fiber grains such as wild rice, rolled oats, and quinoa flakes.

A person with Ulcerative Colitis should also obtain adequate sleep, engage in regular physical exercise each day, and attempt to maintain a healthy social life as much as possible. This will lift one's spirits, enhance one's general health, and aid in the long-term management of the disease.

Because everyone's physiology is different, two persons with Ulcerative Colitis may have distinct trigger foods. You and your doctor can narrow down your personal food triggers by keeping track of what you eat during the day and when digestive problems arise. This is especially beneficial if you are attempting a new diet.

If your Ulcerative Colitis symptoms are worsening, you may realize that eating little meals rather than a large meal makes you feel better. This method can work as long as you eat regularly enough to acquire enough calories and nutrition. Even when they are symptom-free, some people with inflammatory bowel disease find that eating this way helps them control their illness. People with Ulcerative Colitis may also prefer to eat and drink at different times to prevent feeling too full or becoming too full too soon.

Cooking not only allows you to modify the way your food tastes but also allows you to change the physical qualities of the meal to make it simpler to digest. If you are diagnosed with Ulcerative Colitis, you should avoid adding spices, oils, butter, lard, or cheese to your diet since they are difficult to digest and irritate your intestines. The exception is olive oil, which may help reduce the incidence of Ulcerative Colitis in modest amounts, such as those used for cooking. Extra-virgin olive oil, on the other hand, has been proven to have beneficial benefits in several studies, as previously mentioned.

One of the most pleasurable parts of our day is meant to be sitting down to a nice meal. But if you have inflammatory bowel disease, this is not always ideal because what you eat has a major impact on how good or how bad you feel. Eating out at restaurants is the most difficult aspect of managing a diet for many persons with Ulcerative Colitis or any other inflammatory bowel illness. One of the best ideas is to go through the restaurant menu before you go so you can see what you have to choose from and make better decisions. Most restaurants now post their menus online, and some even indicate which items are best for people on special diets, such as low-fat entrees.

Ulcerative Colitis is not caused by food, although it can make it difficult to eat healthily. If spinach, for example, aggravates your symptoms, you may be inclined to avoid all vegetables. However, you would be deficient in nutrition. So make sure to include all of the food categories on your plate. Consider balance rather than extremes.

Flares exhaust you. Anemia, which occurs when your body does not have enough healthy red blood cells, is one cause. You may develop iron deficiency anemia and require iron supplements if you experience long-term, low-level bleeding from your colon's lining or bloody diarrhea. Lean meats, shellfish, spinach, raisins, and fortified breakfast cereals are all good sources of iron. Other alternatives that may be easy on your stomach are egg yolks and artichokes.

If you cannot eat solid foods, smoothies and meal replacement beverages are a wonderful way to acquire nourishment. They are also simple methods to boost nutrients and calories if you are struggling to maintain your weight. Because Ulcerative Colitis makes dehydration more frequent, it is also vital to drink plenty of water and other liquids.

You may be lactose intolerant if dairy makes your symptoms worse. Lactose-free foods, such as hard cheeses and yogurt, can be tried. Lactaid, an enzyme supplement, may also be beneficial. If you must avoid dairy, search for calcium and vitamin D-fortified almond milk and soy cheeses. You will need them since inflammatory bowel disease and its treatment can increase the risk of bone loss.

Broccoli, cauliflower, and beans all produce gas and are difficult to digest. They may also cause diarrhea and cramping. However, they are healthy, so test them well-cooked before putting them on your "No" list. This may solve the issue.

Stick to whole foods and as few processed foods (or none if it is possible). This includes foods such as vegetables, fruits, legumes, and other plant-based foods. It is a good piece of advice to remember that if the food product originated from a machine, it is best not to buy it and consume it.

Ulcerative Colitis is linked with cramps. Eating five to six modest meals each day is one method. Alternatively, have three modest meals and two or three snacks. You can assist prevent discomfort and provide your body a constant supply of nutrients by giving your digestive system fewer quantities to work with.

Keep track of what you eat and how you feel from day to day, whether on paper or on your phone. Look for meals that make you feel nauseous. For a while, stay away from such things. Then, one by one, reintroduce them into your diet to observe how they impact you. Caffeinated and carbonated drinks, as well as spicy and fatty meals, are typical triggers.

Ulcerative Colitis can make it difficult to eat certain foods. So think beyond the box. Even meals that appear to be harmful, such as pizza, may be made to work with a few changes. Lean protein, low-fat dairy, and veggies on a piece of vegetarian pizza are examples of items that include multiple dietary groups. Look for ways to work within your constraints.

Animal products should be avoided or minimized as much as possible. Meats, particularly red meats, are particularly popular. Meats tend to rot in our stomachs as a result of low stomach acidity and poor digestion, generating pus and leading to inflammation, which may be particularly harmful to those with inflammatory bowel illnesses like Ulcerative Colitis. This degradation might lead to an increase in intestinal gas and sluggish digestion.

There is no one-size-fits-all diet for Ulcerative Colitis patients. Consult with your doctor or a nutritionist. They can recommend foods that are both easy to digest and healthy. These professionals will also check to determine if you are deficient in any important nutrients and offer recommendations to ensure you obtain what you require. Also, if you are suffering from any other disease, they will know what your body needs and they can help you manage any possible and unwanted triggers.

It is just as significant how you take your Ulcerative Colitis medicines as it is what you take. For a brief period, your doctor may give steroids or topical medication, but unless your Ulcerative Colitis is light, biologic medicines, which operate on the immune system and help reduce inflammation, are the most common treatment options today. To keep the drug's efficacy, you must take it exactly as directed. There is a considerably increased risk of flare when someone diagnosed with Ulcerative Colitis does not take the recommended medicine at the correct dose. The objective is to persuade the body that the medication is a natural part of them.

4.1 Savory Turmeric Chickpea Oats

Cooking time: 20 minutes

Ingredients

- 1/2 cup rolled oats

- 1/2 cup plant-based milk (soy, almond, oat, or cashew milk, that has not been sweetened)

- 1/2 cup of water

- Add a little pinch of salt

- 1/3 cup of chopped frozen spinach, that is already defrosted (you can also use baby spinach, depends on what you like more)

- 1 tablespoon nutritional yeast

- Add a little pinch of black pepper

- 1/4 teaspoon turmeric

- 1/3 cup precooked chickpeas

Instructions

1. 1.Quick method: In a small dish or saucepan, combine the oats, plant milk, water, salt, and pepper. Refrigerate overnight, covered. In a small pot, bring oats to a boil in the morning. Reduce the heat to a low simmer, add the baby spinach on top of the oats, and

cover the pot to allow the spinach to wilt (this will only take a few minutes).

2. Stir the spinach into the oats fully after it has wilted. (Alternatively, add the frozen, chopped spinach after lowering the heat to low heat and continuing to cook.)

3. Toss in the turmeric. Cook the oats until they're thick and creamy, stirring regularly. Because you soaked the oats overnight, it will just take a few minutes. Add the nutritional yeast, additional salt and/or pepper to taste, and any optional toppings/additions, as well as an extra splash of plant milk if preferred. Serve with chickpeas on top.

(A little) extended method: In a small saucepan, combine the oats, water, plant milk, salt, and pepper and bring to a boil over medium heat. Reduce to low heat and continue to cook as directed above. It'll just take a few minutes longer than soaking the oats. Enjoy!

4.2 Hummus Dip With Creamy Turmeric Sweet Potato

Cooking time: 10 minutes

Ingredients

- 1 peeled and sliced sweet potato (medium)
- 1/2 teaspoon turmeric
- 1/2 teaspoon crushed cumin
- 1/2 teaspoon smoked paprika
- 3 garlic cloves
- 1 tablespoon oil (avocado, if possible)
- 1/2 teaspoon lemon juice
- 1 can rinsed and drained white beans
- 1 tablespoon of tahini
- season with pepper and salt for your taste
- 2 tablespoons extra virgin olive oil

Instructions

1. Preheat the oven to 175 degrees Celsius. Put the sweet potatoes on a baking sheet and mix with the spices and garlic. Bake sweet potatoes for 30-40 minutes, or until they are soft. Allow it to cool before combining with the remaining ingredients (excluding the olive oil) in a food processor. Blend until smooth and creamy, then sprinkle in the olive oil gently while the machine is going. Taste and

adjust seasonings before serving with veggie crudités or pita chips!

4.3 Vegan Turmeric Quinoa Power Bowls

Cooking time: 10 minutes

Ingredients

- 7 potatoes
- chickpeas (15 oz. can)
- 1 tsp paprika
- 1 tsp paprika
- 1 tablespoon of coconut oil
- 1/4 cup quinoa
- add salt and pepper for your taste
- 2 leaves of kale
- 1 tablespoon of extra virgin olive oil
- 1 avocado

Instruction

2. Preheat the oven to 350 degrees Fahrenheit. Using 1/2 of a baking sheet, slice the potatoes into strips and put them flat. Sprinkle 1 tsp turmeric over them and spray/drizzle with coconut oil. Season with salt and pepper to taste. While draining and rinsing the chickpeas, roast for 5 minutes. In a mixing basin, toss the chickpeas with 1 tsp paprika and coat evenly. On the opposite half of the baking sheet, spread the chickpeas. For around 25 minutes, roast the chickpeas and potatoes (or until the potatoes are a little bit soft). 1/2 cup water is used to cook the quinoa. Add 1 tsp turmeric (salt/pepper to season) to the cooked quinoa, stir well, and set aside to cool. Wash the kale leaves and rub the olive oil into them. Divide the leaves amongst the four basins. Cut

the avocado in half and divide it among the four bowls. Serve the quinoa with the roasted chickpeas/potatoes in the bowls!

4.4 Shrimp With Garlic Turmeric And Mango

Cooking time: 20 minutes

Ingredients

- 1 tablespoon of extra virgin olive oil
- 2 limes, cut in half
- 1 tsp salt (kosher)
- 1/8 teaspoon black pepper, ground
- 1 red cabbage head, shredded
- 1 mango
- 1/4 of a tiny red onion, thinly sliced
- 2 tablespoon cilantro, chopped
- 1 pound diced shrimp
- 2 smashed garlic cloves
- 1/4 of turmeric
- 1/4 of cumin
- 1/8 teaspoon crushed red pepper flakes

Instructions

3. Blend1 tablespoon olive oil, the juice of one lime, and 3/4 teaspoon salt and pepper. Then add the cabbage, red onion, mango, and 1 tablespoon fresh cilantro to a mixing bowl. Combine the shrimp, remaining salt, turmeric, crushed red pepper flakes, and cumin in a mixing bowl. Add 1/2 teaspoon olive oil in a large deep nonstick saute pan over medium-high heat, sauté half of the shrimp 1 1/2 to 2

minutes on each side until cooked through and opaque. Set aside, then add the remaining 1/2 teaspoon of oil and the remaining shrimp, and sauté until the shrimp are cooked through and opaque, about 1 minute. Return all of the shrimp to the skillet with the garlic and toss to mix. Remove the shrimp from the heat and mix with cilantro and lime juice. Serve the salad (about 1 1/4 cup) and shrimp on four dishes.

4.5 turmeric Soup with Cauliflower and Kale

Cooking time: 15 minutes

Ingredients

- 1 tablespoon of extra virgin olive oil
- 1 diced onion
- 1 coarsely sliced medium carrot
- 2 celery stalks, finely chopped
- 1 tablespoon turmeric powder
- 2 teaspoons minced garlic (about 4 cloves)
- 1/2 teaspoon ginger powder
- 1/4 teaspoon cayenne pepper, ground
- 1 carton of vegetable broth (32 ounces)
- water, 3–4 cups
- 1 teaspoon salt
- 1 can beans, drained and rinsed
- 3 cups cauliflower florets
- 1 bunch chopped kale
- 1 bunch chopped kale

Instructions

4. Warm the oil in a big saucepan or pot on low. Stir in the onion Cook, stirring occasionally, for 5-7 minutes, or until the onions start to brown. Cook for 3-5 minutes more, or until carrots and celery are softened. Stir in the turmeric,

garlic, ginger, and cayenne until the veggies are well covered. Cook, stirring constantly, for 1 minute or until aromatic. Stir in the broth, water, salt, and pepper until everything is well combined. Bring to a boil, then lower to a low heat setting. Toss in the cauliflower. Cover and cook until cauliflower is soft, about 10-15 minutes. Add the beans, greens, and noodles when the cauliflower is fork soft. Cook until the kale has wilted somewhat. Serve immediately while it is still hot.

4.6 Turmeric Ginger Colada Smoothie

Cooking time: 5 minutes

Ingredients

- 1 inch peeled piece of fresh turmeric (or 1 tsp. dried turmeric)
- 1 inch of peeled fresh ginger
- 1 frozen banana
- 1 cup pineapple chunks (fresh)
- 1 cup of plant-based milk
- a teaspoon of vanilla extract

Instructions

5. Blend the turmeric, ginger, banana, and pineapple until smooth, scraping down the sides of the pitcher as required. Pour in the milk and vanilla extract. Blend until smooth once more.

4.7 Golden Milk High Protein Bites (Healthy, No Baking Needed)

Cooking time: 15 minutes

Ingredients

- 1 3/4 cup gluten-free oat flour
- 1/4 cup coconut flour
- 2 teaspoon sweetener
- 1 tsp turmeric powder
- 1 tsp ginger powder
- 1/2 tsp black pepper
- Optional: 1 tsp cinnamon
- 1/2 cup applesauce, unsweetened
- 1 teaspoon vanilla extract
- 1/4 cup butter
- 1/4 cup maple syrup

Instructions

6. Combine the flour, sugar, and spices in a large mixing basin and stir thoroughly. Heat the nut butter and sticky sweetener together in a microwave-safe bowl or on the stovetop until mixed. Blend in the vanilla extract. Combine the wet mixture and unsweetened applesauce in a large mixing bowl. Depending on the consistency, apply more dairy-free milk or flour until a solid texture is achieved. Form into little bite-sized balls using your palms. Place the balls on a baking sheet or dish and roll them in the optional

granulated sweetener/turmeric combination. To firm up, refrigerate for at least 10 minutes

4.8 Turmeric Rice With Spinach Tofu

Cooking time: 25 minutes

Ingredients

- For the rice:
- 1 cup of brown rice
- 2 cups vegetable broth
- 1/2 teaspoon turmeric
- For the spinach tofu:
- 14 ounce box firm tofu, sliced into squares
- 3 tbsp. olive oil
- 6 cups of spinach
- to taste, freshly grated ginger
- season with salt and pepper to taste.
- choice of dry seasoning – to taste
- lemon juice – to taste, freshly squeezed.
- add sesame seeds to taste

Instructions

7. Put all of the ingredients to a boil in a medium-sized saucepan. Reduce heat to low and cover for 20 minutes, or until water is absorbed. Before serving, fluff. In a deep pan over medium-high heat, heat the olive oil, then add the tofu in a single layer. You may have to cook in batches. Garnish with grated ginger and seasonings to taste. Cook, turning once until lightly browned. It takes about 15 minutes.

Remove the tofu and lay it on a paper towel to absorb any excess liquid. Add one cup of spinach at a time to the same pan until wilted. To taste, season with salt and pepper. To serve you can toss the rice with spinach on one side and tofu on the other in a serving dish. Or serve with sesame seeds and a hefty squeeze of lemon juice on top of the spinach.

4.9 CHICKEN WITH TURMERIC HONEY MUSTARD

Cooking time: 35 minutes

Ingredients

- 6 – 8 bone-in, skin-on chicken thighs (or however you prefer)

- For the rub:

- 1 tablespoon of extra virgin olive oil

- 1 tsp turmeric powder

- 1 teaspoon powdered mustard

- a pinch of salt and pepper

- To make the honey-mustard sauce, combine all of the next ingredients in a mixing bowl:

- 3 tablespoon mustard (whole grain)

- 3 tablespoon mustard (Dijon)

- honey, 3 tablespoons

- 2 tablespoon chicken stock

- salt and pepper (season to taste)

Instructions

8. Preheat the oven to 375 degrees Fahrenheit. Dry the chicken thighs. Combine all of the rub ingredients and massage them all over the chicken thighs. Set aside the honey-mustard sauce ingredients after whisking them together. On the stove, heat a big oven-safe pan with a heavy bottom. When the pan is hot, drizzle in enough oil to just cover the

surface. Add the chicken thighs, skin side down, when it begins to shimmer.

4.10 Blueberry Galette (Gluten-Free)

Cooking time: 60-70 minutes

Ingredients

- For the pastry:
- 2 1/4 cup of cashew flour
- 1/4 cup plus 3 teaspoons arrowroot powder
- 1 tablespoon flour (coconut)
- a quarter teaspoon of salt
- 1/4 cup maple syrup, undiluted
- 5 tablespoons unsalted cold grass-fed butter
- For the filling:
- 2 cups of blueberries
- 1 teaspoon of maple syrup
- 1 tablespoon sugar (coconut)
- 2 tablespoons powdered arrowroot
- 1 1/2 teaspoons lemon juice (it is better to use fresh lemon juice)
- zest of 1 lemon
- Egg wash:
- 1 egg yolk (large, if possible)
- 1 tablespoon of full-fat milk (coconut or any plant-based kind)

Instructions

9. Combine the cashew flour, arrowroot, coconut flour, and sea salt in a food processor and pulse for 15 seconds, or until mixed. Process for 15 seconds, or until the maple syrup is mixed and crumbly. Add 1 tablespoon cold butter at a time, pulsing the food processor a few times between each addition until the butter is pea-sized and the dough starts to come together. Pack the dough into a tight ball and flatten it into a disc with your hands. Wrap it firmly in plastic wrap and put it in the refrigerator for 4 hours to cool. Preheat the oven to 325°F once the dough has chilled. Place the dough on a flat surface between two big pieces of parchment paper. Roll out the dough into a 12-inch-diameter circle that is about 1/2-inch thick. Place the dough, paper, and baking sheet on a baking sheet. In a mixing dish, add all of the filling ingredients and whisk gently until well mixed. Fill the middle of the rolled-out pastry with the filling. Fold up the sides of the dough to leave about 2 inches of pastry overhanging the filling's exterior border. Combine the egg yolk and coconut milk in a mixing bowl. Apply a little coat of egg wash to the top of the puff pastry with a pastry brush. Preheat the oven to 350°F and bake the galette for 45 minutes, or until golden brown on top. It is best to serve the dish while it is still warm.

4.11 Broiled Salmon

Cooking time: 30 minutes

Ingredients

- 4 fillets of salmon
- 2 tablespoons extra virgin olive oil
- 2 teaspoons of salt
- 1–2 lemons, sliced

Instructions

10. Preheat the broiler to high. Use parchment paper or lightly oil a pan or dish. Salmon fillets should be patted dry and properly seasoned with salt and olive oil. Place on the top shelf of the oven for 10 minutes for every inch of thickness of the fillets (for crispiness). When ready to serve, garnish with cut lemon slices and offer pieces for each individual to add juice as needed.

4.12 Chocolate Candies With Coconut Oil

Cooking time: 20 minutes

Ingredients

- 1/2 cup of coconut oil

- 1/4 cup of cocoa powder

- 2 tablespoons raw organic honey (adjust according to taste, you can also use your favorite kind of honey)

- 1 tsp vanilla extract (this is optional, but it is best if you use pure vanilla extract)

Instructions

11. Melt the coconut oil in a small saucepan. Heat the oil just enough to melt it without overheating it. Microwave for 15 seconds on high, then whisk and repeat if necessary. At body temperature, coconut oil converts to a liquid form, thus it doesn't need to be heated any higher. This is because the hotter the liquid, the longer it will take to cool, allowing the mixture more time to separate once in the mold. If you have a blender, mix the coconut oil and honey and process until smooth. If you don't have a blender, whisk everything together thoroughly. Blend or whisk in the cocoa powder until it is completely smooth. Fill an ice cube pan or a tiny muffin dish halfway with the mixture (silicone ones work best). Refrigerate or freeze for 30 minutes to cool. Note that the amount of time required varies depending on how hot the coconut oil was when you began. These can be set in as little as 15 minutes if the oil has just reached the melting point. After you have made them, store them in the freezer or refrigerator since they will melt quickly in warm weather. This recipe makes around 25 tiny chocolates.

4.13 Oat Soup With Beef

Cooking time: 15 minutes

Ingredients

- 1pound ground beef (lean)
- 1/2 teaspoon pepper, freshly ground, divided
- 4 tablespoon of extra virgin olive oil (split)
- 1 medium coarsely chopped onion
- 1/2 – 1lb spinach, grinded
- 1 big shredded carrot
- 1 tablespoon fresh thyme, chopped (or ground)
- a cup of oats
- 4 cups beef broth (low sodium)
- 14 teaspoon salt 1 cup water
- 1-2 tablespoons of red-wine vinegar (taste to adjust)

Instructions

12. Bring a pot of water to a boil with 3-4 cups of water. Boil the oats in a separate pot. Reduce heat to low and cook for 30 minutes or longer. (Refer to the oats box for specific cooking instructions.) 1/4 teaspoon pepper should be sprinkled over the beef. In an oven, heat 2 tablespoons of oil over medium heat. Cook, turning often until the meat is browned on both sides, approximately 2 minutes. Place in a mixing basin. Cook, stirring occasionally until the remaining 2 tablespoons oil has evaporated and the onion has begun to soften approximately 2 minutes. Cook for another 2

minutes, stirring constantly. Toss in the spinach. Cook, stirring occasionally until the veggies are beginning to brown, about 1 to 2 minutes. Bring to a simmer the oats, broth, water, salt, and the remaining 1/4 teaspoon pepper. Reduce the heat to keep the mixture at a low simmer for about 15 minutes. Return the meat to the saucepan, along with any collected juices, and cook through for 1 to 2 minutes. Remove the pan from the heat and add the vinegar to taste. These may be kept in the refrigerator for two weeks or frozen for several months. Remove the bars from the freezer for about 20 minutes before serving if you are storing them.

4.14 SPINACH SOUP

Cooking time: 15 minutes

Ingredients

- 1 tablespoon olive oil (extra virgin)
- 14 tsp turmeric,
- onion (coarsely chopped)
- 4 cups stock (vegetable or chicken) (sugar and wheat-free)
- chopped scallions (green onions)
- 1/3 cup of oats
- 1 pound of baby spinach (washed, stems removed)
- 2 cups plain yogurt (low fat or nonfat)
- 2 garlic cloves, smashed
- salt and pepper to your own taste

Instructions

13. In a large saucepan, heat the olive oil and sauté the onion until tender. Cook for approximately a minute after adding the turmeric. Add the stock, scallions, oats, salt, and pepper to taste. Cook for 15 minutes on low heat. Take cautious not to overcook the food. Cut the spinach into small pieces. Cook for another five minutes in the pan.

14. Side note: If you are serving the soup hot, stir in the yogurt and garlic and gradually reheat the soup so the yogurt doesn't curdle. Using a blender or a food processor, puree the mixture. If you wish to serve the soup cold, let it cool

somewhat before adding the yogurt and garlic and puréeing.

4.15 Oat Pancakes With Banana And Almond

Cooking time: 10 minutes

Ingredients

- 1 cup oats, rolled
- 1/4 cup of almonds (or around a third of a cup of almond meal)
- 1/2 teaspoon of cinnamon
- 1/2 teaspoon of nutmeg
- 1/2 teaspoon of baking soda
- 1 banana, medium
- 1 tablespoon of vinegar
- 1 tsp vanilla extract (pure)
- 1 egg
- 3/4 cup almond or soy milk, unsweetened

Instructions

1. In a food processor or blender, grind the oats (and almonds if preparing almond flour from whole almonds). Combine the ground oats, almond flour, cinnamon, nutmeg, and baking soda in a mixing dish. Mash the banana in a separate dish. Then add the vinegar, vanilla, egg, and almond or soy milk, whisking constantly. To make the batter, combine the dry ingredients with the wet ones. Using canola oil, gently coat a nonstick griddle over medium heat. Pour approximately a quarter cup of batter onto the griddle. Cook for 3-4 minutes, until the edges, begin to brown slightly and a few bubbles appear. Flip. You can top the

pancakes with whatever you prefer. Feel free to mix tastes and enjoy!

4.16 Scrambled Tofu

Cooking time: 20 minutes

Ingredients

- 1 pound drained and crumbled extra-firm tofu
- 12ounces tomato sauce or paste (whatever you prefer more)
- 1 teaspoon turmeric
- 1/2 cup of diced zucchini
- 1/2 cup of diced onions
- 1/2 cup of diced mushrooms
- 1 tablespoon of extra virgin olive oil
- sauce with a hot kick (as tolerated)
- Soy cheese (shredded)

Instructions

1. In a large pan, heat about 1 tablespoon of olive oil. Onions and turmeric should be sautéed till transparent. Gradually add tofu and other veggies. Cook until the tofu is slightly browned and the veggies are tender. Drain any excess water. Mix salsa well. Hot sauce can be used to taste. If desired, top with cheese.

4.17. Crackers With Herbs

Cooking time: 20 minutes

Ingredients

- 3 ½ cups of flour (almond)
- 2 tablespoons coarsely chopped rosemary (fresh)
- 2 tablespoons fresh thyme, coarsely chopped
- 2 tablespoons of olive oil (extra virgin is better)
- 2 eggs (large, if possible)
- 1 teaspoon of sea salt

Instructions

1. Preheat the oven to 350 degrees Fahrenheit. 2 big baking sheets should be set aside. 3 parchment paper sheets, cut to the size of the baking sheets. Combine the almond flour, salt, rosemary, and thyme in a large mixing basin. Whisk together the olive oil and eggs in a medium mixing basin. Combine the wet components and stir them into the almond flour mixture until everything is well mixed. Divide the dough into two equal halves. Roll one piece of dough between two pieces of parchment paper to a thickness of 1/16 inch. Remove the top piece of parchment paper and place the bottom piece of parchment on the baking sheet with the rolled-out dough. Carry on with the remaining dough piece in the same manner. Using a knife or a pizza cutter, cut the dough into 2-inch squares. Preheat oven to 350°F and bake for 12-15 minutes, or until gently brown. (If you want your crackers to be even crisper, throw them back in for another 15 minutes once they've cooled.) Allow 30 minutes for the crackers to cool on the baking pan before serving.

4.18 FLAX BARS WITH WALNUTS

Cooking time: 15 minutes

Ingredients

- 3 tablespoons walnut oil (you can also use canola oil)
- 1/3 cup raw honey (you can use less if you want)
- 2 organic eggs
- 3/4 cups of diced walnuts
- 2 teaspoons of vanilla extract (pure)
- 1 cup of chia seeds (oats can be an option, too)
- 1/2 teaspoon of baking powder
- 2/3 cups of grounded flaxseeds

Instructions

1. Preheat the oven to 350 degrees Fahrenheit. Combine the first seven ingredients (oil to wheat germ) in a mixing bowl. Combine the oats or Chia seeds with the baking powder and incorporate them into the whipped mixture. Pour the mixture into an 8-inch shallow square pan that has been oiled. Preheat oven to 350°F and bake for 25 minutes, or until firm to the touch. Serve by cutting into squares.

4.19. Avocado Salsa With Mango

Cooking time: 5 minutes

Ingredients

- 2 tablespoons of olive oil (extra virgin is better)
- 1 tiny red onion
- 1/2 cilantro leaves, fresh and diced
- 1 avocado, sliced
- 1 mango (large and sliced)
- 2 garlic cloves, diced (this is optional)
- 1 jalapeño pepper, minced (also optional, if you do use it, remove the seeds)
- 1/4 cup of lime juice, freshly squeezed (you can also use lemon juice)

Instructions

1. Combine the mango, onion, avocado, cilantro, garlic, jalapeño, and lime juice in a mixing bowl. Serve with fish, other entrees, or as a great snack on its own!

4.20. Broccoli With Sesame Seeds

Cooking time: 20 minutes

Ingredients

- 1 ½ pound of fresh broccoli (you can also use frozen)
- 1 tablespoon of extra virgin olive oil
- 2 tablespoons of sesame seeds
- 1 tablespoon of freshly squeezed lemon juice
- 1 tablespoon of soy sauce
- 2 teaspoons of raw honey

Instructions

1. Place broccoli in a vegetable steamer over boiling water and cut it into big pieces. Cover and steam for 5-6 minutes, or until the vegetables are brilliant green. Drain the broccoli and set it in a serving dish. In a small saucepan, heat the oil over medium heat. Cook until the sesame seeds are gently toasted. Bring the lemon juice, tamari, and honey to a boil. Remove the pan from the heat and pour the sauce over the broccoli, tossing to coat. And it is ready to taste.

4.21 SEASONED CHICKEN (baked)

Cooking time: 35 minutes

Ingredients

- 2/3 pound cut-up chicken (skinless)
- 6 oz. tomato puree
- 1/4 cup of vinegar
- 1/2 teaspoon celery seeds
- 1/4 teaspoon mustard powder
- 1/8 teaspoon cinnamon powder
- 1/8 teaspoon clove powder
- 2 cups orange juice (chicken broth with low sodium is also an option)
- 2 tablespoons minced onion
- 1/4 teaspoon salt

Instructions

1. Place the chicken in a baking dish that has been gently oiled. In a pan, combine the remaining ingredients and bring to a boil. Reduce heat to low and cook for 5 minutes. Pour the sauce over the chicken. Bake for 1 hour or until done, basting regularly at 350 degrees. Taste to know when the chicken is done and ready to eat.

4.22 BREAD WITH ZUCCHINI

Cooking time: 35 minutes

Ingredients

- 2 cups almond flour (rinsed)
- 1/2 tablespoon of salt
- 1 teaspoon cinnamon powder
- 1/4 cup of canola oil
- 1/2 cup honey (local honey is preferable)
- 2 eggs (large, if possible)
- 1 cup of zucchini (grated)
- 1/2 teaspoon baking soda
- 1/2 cup coarsely chopped pecans
- 1/4 cup dried currants (this is an optional ingredient)

Instructions

1. Preheat the oven to 350 degrees Fahrenheit. 2 mini loaf pans, lightly greased with grapeseed oil and dusted with almond flour. Combine the almond flour, salt, baking soda, and cinnamon in a large mixing basin. Whisk together the grapeseed oil, honey, and eggs in a medium mixing basin. After completely combining the almond flour mixture with the wet ingredients, fold in the zucchini, pecans, and currants. Fill the pans halfway with batter. Bake on the bottom rack of the oven for 50 to 60 minutes, or until a knife inserted in the middle comes out clean. Allow 1 hour for the bread to cool in the pans before serving.

4.23 Mushrooms With Green Beans

Cooking time: 20 minutes

Ingredients

- 6 tablespoon of extra virgin olive
- 8 oz. mushrooms, fresh (remove and slice the stems)
- 3 shallots, sliced
- 2 cloves garlic
- 2 pounds of slender green beans
- 1/2 cup of broth (chicken or vegetable)
- For seasoning, use ground pepper or sea salt.

Instructions

1. In a large skillet, heat the oil over medium-high heat 3 tablespoons of extra virgin olive oil When the pan is heated, add the mushrooms and cook until they are soft. Place mushrooms in a mixing basin. In the same skillet, add the remaining 3 tablespoons of oil. Garlic and shallots, chopped. Still for a couple minutes, or until the vegetables are soft. Toss in the green beans to coat. Pour half a cup of broth over the green bean mixture if using frozen beans. Cover and cook until the liquid has evaporated and the green beans are tender but still crunchy. Cooked mushrooms should be added now. Season the meal your own taste and the meal and it is ready to eat!

4.24 VEGETABLE SMOOTHIE

Cooking time: 5 minutes

Ingredients

- 1/2 cup ice water
- 1/2 red bell pepper (or a color of your choice)
- 1 carrot
- 1/2 kale leaves
- 1 stalk of celery
- 1/2 green or red apple
- 8 almonds (whole)
- a thin slice of ginger (fresh or frozen)
- 5-6 ice cubes
- *You can also add some frozen fruit like grapes or mango.

Instructions

1. Combine all the ingredients and mix them in a blender. This is the perfect morning smoothie. It is delicious and healthy, which means you will have energy for many hours.

4.25 CARROT SOUP WITH GINGER

Cooking time: 20 minutes

Ingredients

- 1/2 of chopped butternut squash
- 1 pound of peeled and diced carrots
- 2 cups of water
- 15 thin slices of peeled ginger
- 1 chopped onion
- 2 cups of water minced garlic cloves
- season with salt and pepper to taste
- a pinch of cinnamon

Instructions

1. Sauté a couple garlic cloves and a diced onion in olive oil in a big saucepan, then add 2 cups water and butternut squash (chopped). Add the carrots and fresh ginger while it's simmering. Season with salt, pepper, and a few shakes of cinnamon to taste. Allow for at least 20 minutes of cooking time. In a food processor or blender, puree the entire mixture until smooth. If necessary, add a splash of boiling water to the blender to achieve the correct consistency, but be cautious not to overdo it. This soup is a purée, which means it's thick and creamy. If desired, a dab of butter can be added to the bowl and mixed before serving.

4.26 Chocolate Pudding With Avocado

Cooking time: 5 minutes

Ingredients

- 2 avocados (ripe)
- 1/2 cup coconut milk
- 6 tablespoons cocoa powder (not sweetened)
- 5 tablespoons of honey
- 1 teaspoon cinnamon powder
- 1 teaspoon vanilla extract
- 1/2 teaspoon of salt

Instructions

1. In a blender, mix all of the ingredients until smooth. And that is it. For serving you can use more fruits and this can also be a dessert topping.

4.27 Cake With Coffee And Cinnamon

Cooking time: 35 minutes

Ingredients

- For the cake:
- 2 ½ cups flour (preferably almond)
- 1/2 tablespoon baking soda
- 1/4 teaspoon salt
- 1/2 cup chopped walnuts
- 1/2 cup currants, dried
- 1/4 cup of canola oil
- 1/4 cup honey
- 2 eggs (large)
- For the topping:
- 2 teaspoons cinnamon powder
- 2 tablespoons of oil (canola)
- 1/2 cup chopped almonds
- 1/4 cup of honey

Instructions

1. Preheat the oven to 350 degrees Fahrenheit. Dust an 8-inch square baking dish with almond flour after brushing it with canola oil. In a large mixing basin, combine the almond flour, salt, baking soda, walnuts, and currants. Whisk together the canola oil, honey, and eggs in a medium mixing basin. Combine the wet components and stir them into the

almond flour mixture until everything is well mixed. Put the batter into the baking dish and spread it out. In a mixing bowl, combine the cinnamon, canola oil, honey, and almonds to form the topping. Over the cake batter, sprinkle the topping. Bake the cake for 25-35 minutes, or until a toothpick inserted in the center comes out clean. Allow 1 hour for the cake to cool in the pan before serving.

4.28 Smoothie With Frozen Fruits

Cooking time: 5 minutes

Ingredients

- 1/3 cup of orange juice
- 1/3 cup of frozen blueberries
- 10 frozen grapes
- 2 tablespoons plant-based yogurt

Instructions

1. In a blender, combine all ingredients until they reach the required consistency. Add a tiny quantity of ice halfway through the blending cycle for a colder smoothie.

4.29 Apple Muffins With Cinnamon

Cooking time: 25 minutes

Ingredients

- 1/2 teaspoon salt

- 1 teaspoon cinnamon powder

- 2 1/4 cup almond flour

- 1/4 cup of oil (canola)

- 1/2 cup of honey

- 1 egg

- 1 tablespoon vanilla extract

- 2 apples (peeled and diced)

- 1/2 teaspoon baking soda

Instructions

1. Preheat the oven to 350 degrees Fahrenheit. Paper liners should be used to line 10 muffin cups. Combine the almond flour, salt, baking soda, and cinnamon in a large mixing basin. Whisk together the canola oil, honey, egg, and vanilla extract in a medium mixing bowl. After completely mixing the wet ingredients into the almond flour mixture, fold in the apples. Fill the muffin cups halfway with batter. Bake for 25-30 minutes, or until golden brown on top and a toothpick inserted into the center comes out clean. Allow 30 minutes for the muffins to cool in the pan before serving.

4.30 Banana Cake With Cranberries

Cooking time: 30 minutes

Ingredients

- 1/2 cup almond flour
- 1 ½ rolled oats
- 1 teaspoon of baking soda
- 1/2 teaspoon salt
- 2-3 ripe bananas, mashed
- 1/2 cup of coconut oil
- 1 teaspoon lemon extract
- 3 eggs

Instructions

1. Combine all ingredients, along with 1/3 cup cranberries, and pour into a pan that has been lightly oiled. Preheat oven to 350°F and bake for 30-35 minutes. You shall leave the cake to cool for an hour or two before serving.

4.31 Cucumber Salad

Cooking time: 10 minutes

Ingredients

- 1 tablespoon vinegar
- 1/4 teaspoon of raw honey
- 1 cucumber, peeled and cut
- 1/4 finely sliced red onion
- 1 finely sliced carrot
- add cayenne pepper to taste
- season with salt and freshly ground pepper to taste

Instructions

1. Combine the vinegar, honey, and a pinch of cayenne pepper in a mixing bowl. Add salt and pepper to taste. Toss in the cucumber, purple onion, and carrots to coat. Refrigerate until ready to serve.

4.32 Red Onions With Lime

Cooking time: 15 minutes

Ingredients

- 3 cups red onions, chopped
- 1 seeded and chopped Anaheim pepper
- 2 limes, freshly squeezed
- 1 tablespoon fresh cilantro, diced
- 1/8 teaspoon of chili powder (optional)
- 1/4 tablespoon of cumin powder

Instructions

1. Combine all the ingredients into a bowl and it is ready to serve.
2. You can also add some other ingredients if you feel like it.

4.33 Spinach Smoothie

Cooking time: 5 minutes

Ingredients

- 1 cup of pineapple juice
- 2 cups baby spinach
- 1/3 cup mint leaves
- 1 teaspoon lemon juice, fresh
- 1 tablespoon honey
- 1/2 frozen banana
- 1 small diced cucumber
- 3 ice cubes

Instructions

1. Pulse the ice in the mixer to smash it. Add the spinach, mint, lemon, and pineapple juice and honey; pause to break up the greens, then mix for 20 seconds to 1 minute, depending on your blender. Blend in the cucumber and banana for approximately 45 seconds, or until the mixture is thick and moves smoothly in the blender jar.

4.34 Pineapple Smoothie With Kale

Cooking time: 5 minutes

Ingredients

- 1 ½ cup of coconut milk
- 2 cups of kale leaves
- 1 tablespoon fresh lime juice
- 1 1/2 cups frozen pineapple
- 1/2 frozen banana
- ice cubes (optional)

Instructions

1. Pulse the ice in the mixer to smash it. Combine the coconut milk, kale, and lime juice to break up the greens, then blend to liquefy the solids, first on medium and progressively increasing to high. Blend in the pineapple and banana for approximately 45 seconds, or until the mixture is consistent, thick, and moves smoothly in the blender jar, then serve.

4.35 Chips

Cooking time: 20 minutes

Ingredients

- 2 carrots
- 1 beet
- 1 knob celery
- olive oil (if possible extra virgin)
- salt

Instructions

1. Carrots, beets, and celeriac root should be peeled and sliced into paper-thin slices. Pour 12 to 1 inch of olive oil into a big wok or deep frying pan and heat until it begins to crackle. Place the chips in the pan with the hot oil and cook them. To absorb the extra oil from the chips, place a paper towel on a plate. If preferred, season with salt and serve right away.

4.36 Lime Crackers

Cooking time: 20 minutes

Ingredients

- 2 cups of cheese (non-dairy)
- 1 cups flour
- 3 tablespoons of water
- 1/4 cup of extra virgin olive oil
- 1/4 teaspoon powdered garlic
- 1/4 teaspoon salt
- 1/8 teaspoon powdered turmeric
- 1/2 teaspoon lime zest
- 2 teaspoons of lime or lemon juice

Instructions

1. Preheat the oven to 350 degrees Fahrenheit. A baking tray should be greased. In a mixing dish, combine all of the ingredients. Form into a ball and chill for 15 minutes or until firm. Drop tiny rounds of dough onto the baking pan, properly spaced apart. Flatten the dough circles onto the tray with your hands. Place the crackers in the oven and bake for about 15 minutes, or until golden brown. Allow time for cooling.

4.37 TOMATO SAUCE

Cooking time: 25 minutes

Ingredients

- 4 tablespoons olive oil (extra virgin)
- 1 chopped onion
- 3 diced tomatoes
- 1 tablespoon mashed tomatoes
- season with salt and pepper to taste

Instructions

1. Cook onion in olive oil in a large pan over medium heat until transparent. Cook, stirring constantly until the liquid thickens. Combine the puree, salt, and pepper in a mixing bowl. Reduce heat to low and continue to cook for another 15 minutes, or until the sauce is rich and thick.

4.38 TORTILLAS

Cooking time: 10 minutes

Ingredients

- 1 cup oat flour (gluten-free)
- 1 tablespoon spice mix
- 1/2 cup water

Instructions

1. Combine the flour and spices in a small bowl. After adding the water, check the consistency. The dough should be pliable but not moist, and it should mold into shapes easily. As you mix, the dough will readily form a ball. If required, adjust the consistency with a little more flour or water. Pinch off golf ball-sized balls of dough. Toss them in a little more flour to make sure they're well-coated. Knead each ball slightly before patting or rolling it into a flat circle approximately. Repeat with the remaining dough. Preheat a griddle or a large frying pan. There is no need to use oil. Cook each tortilla for a few minutes on each side in the heated pan. Tortillas should get a light brown color and seem dry. Allow cooling on wire racks.

4.39 BREAD (Paleo)

Cooking time: 20 minutes

Ingredients

- 2 cups almond flour
- 2 tablespoons of coconut flour
- 1/4 cup flax meal (golden)
- 1/4 teaspoon sea salt
- 1/2 tablespoon baking soda
- 5 eggs
- 1 tablespoon oil (coconut)
- 1 tablespoon honey
- 1 tablespoon vinegar

Instructions

1. In a food processor, combine almond flour, coconut flour, flax, salt, and baking soda. Combine the ingredients in a blender and pulse until smooth. In a food processor, combine the eggs, oil, honey, and vinegar. Transfer the batter to a loaf pan. Preheat oven to 350°F and bake for 30 minutes. Allow 2 hours to cool in the pan and then it is ready to serve.

4.40 CHICKEN NUGGETS

Cooking time: 25 minutes

Ingredients

- 1 ½ pound chicken breast (boneless and skinless)

- 1 cup flour (almond)

- 1/2 teaspoon salt

- 1/2 teaspoon pepper

- 2 eggs

- 1/2 cup of low-fat yogurt

- For frying, you can use extra virgin olive oil

Instructions

1. Chicken should be cut into nugget-sized pieces. In a medium mixing bowl, sift the almond flour. Season with salt and pepper. In a separate dish, whisk together the eggs and yogurt. Stir until everything is fully combined. Dredge the chicken in the almond flour until uniformly covered after dipping it in the egg mixture. Place the nuggets on a dish and set them aside. Preheat the frying pan to medium-high heat. Add roughly a half-inch of oil to the pan. In the pan, arrange a single layer of chicken. Cook each side for about 3 minutes. The crust should have a golden brown color to it. You may check if the chicken is cooked through by cutting open one of the nuggets. To absorb any excess oil, place the nuggets on paper towels. As much as possible,

allow them to dry. Continue until all of the nuggets have been fried.

4.41 Baked Chickpeas

Cooking time: 20 minutes

Ingredients

- 1 can of chickpeas (drained)
- 2 tablespoons olive oil
- cayenne pepper (an option)
- garlic powder
- curry powder

Instructions

1. Preheat the oven to 230 degrees C. To dry chickpeas, blot them with a paper towel. Toss chickpeas with olive oil in a mixing bowl, then season with garlic salt, cayenne pepper, or curry powder, if using. Bake for 30 to 40 minutes, until golden and crispy, on a baking sheet. To avoid scorching, keep a close eye on the last few minutes. Let it cool down a little and then it is ready.

4.42 Banana Bars

Cooking time: 15 minutes

Ingredients

- 2 ripe bananas (mashed)
- 2 cups oats (uncooked)
- 1/2 cup non-dairy milk (unsweetened)
- 1 egg
- 2 tablespoons of olive oil
- 1/2 teaspoon vanilla extract
- 2 tablespoon honey
- a hint of salt
- 1 to 2 cups chopped nuts and dried fruit

Instructions

1. Preheat the oven to 375 degrees Fahrenheit. In a mixing dish, combine all of the ingredients and stir thoroughly. Place the batter on a greased cookie sheet, pat it down, and shape it into rough bars that are slightly flat. Depending on whether you want soft or crispy bars, bake for 20 to 30 minutes. Let the bars cool off and they are ready to serve.

4.43 Paprika Crackers

Cooking time: 25 minutes

Ingredients

- 3 cups almond flour

- 1 teaspoon salt

- 1/2 cup chopped pecans

- 1 tablespoon ground paprika

- 1/2 teaspoon ground cumin

- 2 tablespoons oil

- 2 eggs

- 1 teaspoon zest of lemon

Instructions

1. Preheat the oven to 350 degrees Fahrenheit. 2 big baking sheets should be set aside. 3 parchment paper sheets, cut to the size of the baking sheets Combine the almond flour, salt, pecans, paprika, and cumin in a large mixing basin. Whisk together the canola oil, eggs, and lemon zest in a medium mixing basin. Combine the wet components and stir them into the almond flour mixture until everything is well mixed. Divide the dough into two equal halves. Roll one piece of dough between two pieces of parchment paper to a thickness of 1/16 inch. Remove the top piece of parchment paper and place the bottom piece of parchment on the baking sheet with the rolled-out dough. Carry on with the remaining dough piece in the same manner. Using a knife or a pizza cutter, cut the dough into 2-inch squares. Preheat oven to 350°F and bake for 12-15 minutes, or until gently

brown. Allow 30 minutes for the crackers to cool on the baking pan before serving.

4.44 Onion Sticks

Cooking time: 20 minutes

Ingredients

- 3 egg
- 2 cups flour
- 2 garlic cloves
- 2 tablespoons cilantro, fresh and diced
- 1/8 teaspoon baking powder
- 1/3 cup onion, diced
- 1/4 teaspoon salt
- 1/4 teaspoon black pepper

Instructions

1. Preheat the oven to 350 degrees Fahrenheit. Canola oil should be used to grease a baking pan. Whisk the egg whites in a medium-sized mixing basin until stiff. Remove from the equation. Combine the garlic, onion, salt, pepper, baking powder, fresh cilantro, and almond flour in a separate bowl. Fold the egg whites in slowly. Moisture should be present in the dough, but it should not be sticky. Form dough balls 12 inches in diameter and roll them between your palms to form long strands (sticks). Place the rolled sticks on the baking tray, spacing them out evenly. Place the sticks in the oven and bake for 20 to 30 minutes, or until golden brown.

4.45 Chia Pudding

Cooking time: 10 minutes

Ingredients

- 1 cup vanilla almond milk
- 1 cup low-fat yogurt
- 2 tablespoon honey
- 1 teaspoon vanilla extract
- a pinch of salt
- 1/4 cup chia seeds
- *For the topping, you can use mango puree or peaches.

Instructions

1. Stir together all of the ingredients thoroughly and store them in an airtight jar. Make sure the chia seeds are spread equally. Refrigerate for at least one night.

4.46 CARROT CAKE

Cooking time: 35 minutes

Ingredients

- 3 cups almond flour
- 1 teaspoon baking soda
- 2 tablespoons salt
- 1 tablespoon cinnamon powder
- 1 teaspoon nutmeg powder
- 1/4 cup oil
- 1/2 cup honey
- 5 eggs
- 3 cups carrots, diced
- 1 cup raisins
- 1 cup diced walnuts

Instructions

1. Preheat the oven to 325 degrees Fahrenheit. Canola oil and almond flour are used to grease two 9-inch cake pans. Combine the almond flour, salt, baking soda, cinnamon, and nutmeg in a large mixing basin. Whisk together the canola oil, honey, and eggs in a medium mixing basin. Combine the wet components and stir them into the almond flour mixture until everything is well mixed. Combine the carrots, raisins, and walnuts in a mixing bowl. Scoop the batter into the cake pans that have been prepared. Bake for 40 minutes. Put a toothpick in the center, if it is clean, then

it is ready. Allow 1 hour for the cake to cook in the pans before serving.

4.47 PEAR SMOOTHIE

Cooking time: 5 minutes

Ingredients

- 1 banana, ripe and sliced
- 1 pear, diced
- 1 teaspoon ginger
- 3 tablespoons honey
- 1/4 cup almond milk
- 1/4 cup yogurt

Instructions

1. Combine all the ingredients and mix them in a blender. You can add some ice cubes if you want more fresh and cold drink.

4.48 Spinach Quiche

Cooking time: 25 minutes

Ingredients

- 1 tablespoon olive oil

- 1 chopped onion

- 10 ounces of frozen spinach

- 5 eggs

- 3 cups non-dairy cheese

- 1/4 teaspoon salt

- 1/8 teaspoon black pepper

Instructions

1. Preheat the oven to 350 degrees Fahrenheit. Grease a 9-inch pie tin lightly. In a skillet, heat the oil over medium-high heat. Cook, stirring occasionally until onions are tender. Stir the spinach regularly and simmer until all of the liquid has evaporated. Combine eggs, cheese, salt, and pepper in a large mixing basin. Stir in the spinach mixture until everything is well combined. Scoop into the pie pan that has been prepared. Bake for 30 minutes in a preheated oven until the eggs have set. Allow it to cool before serving.

4.49. Toast (French)

Cooking time: 15 minutes

Ingredients

- 1/4 cup non-dairy milk
- 2 tablespoons honey
- 4 eggs
- 1 teaspoon vanilla extract
- 1/4 teaspoon salt
- 1/2 teaspoon cinnamon
- 8-half inch slices of bread
- 2 tablespoons oil

Instructions

1. Whisk together the coconut milk, honey, eggs, vanilla extract, salt, and cinnamon in a medium mixing bowl until well mixed. Fill a 13 by 9-inch baking dish halfway with the mixture and soak the bread slices for 5 minutes on each side. In a skillet, heat the canola oil over medium-high heat. Cook the bread slices for 3 to 5 minutes per side in the oil, until golden brown. Place the French toast on a serving dish. Repeat the process until all of the slices have been completed.

4.50 Pancakes

Cooking time: 15 minutes

Ingredients

- 2 eggs
- 1/4 cup honey
- 1 tablespoon vanilla extract
- 1/4 cup water
- 1 ½ cup flour
- 1/2 teaspoon salt
- 1/2 teaspoon baking soda
- 2 tablespoons oil

Instructions

1. Combine the eggs, honey, vanilla extract, and water in a blender and mix on high for about 1 minute, or until smooth. Blend in the almond flour, salt, and baking soda until well mixed. In a large skillet, heat the canola oil over medium-low heat. For each pancake, pour 1 heaping spoonful of batter into the skillet. Cook until tiny bubbles appear on the surface of each pancake, then flip each pancake as the bubbles begin to open. Transfer to a platter after thoroughly cooked.

4.51 Banana Bread

Cooking time: 35 minutes

Ingredients

- 4 mashed bananas
- 4 tablespoons butter
- 1 teaspoon vanilla extract
- 1 teaspoon baking soda
- 3 cups flour
- 3/4 cup honey
- 4 eggs

Instructions

1. Preheat the oven to 300 degrees Fahrenheit. Line the bottoms of two 1.5-quart loaf pans with parchment paper. Alternatively, muffin pans might be lined with muffin liners. In a food processor, combine all of the ingredients and process until smooth. Fill the loaf pans halfway with batter and bake for 50 minutes, or until the bread is light golden brown. Only bake for 30 minutes if you're preparing muffins.

4.52 Salad With Fruit And Lime Yogurt

Cooking time: 10 minutes

Ingredients

- 1 ripe melon, diced
- 1 pint of strawberries
- 2 mangoes, diced
- 2 bananas, diced
- 2 cup plant-based yogurt
- 2 tablespoons honey
- 1 teaspoon lime zest

Instructions

1. Toss the fruit with the lime juice in a large mixing basin. Allow for 15 minutes of resting time, stirring regularly. Combine yogurt, honey, lime zest, and juice in a small mixing dish and whisk well. Cover it and let it chill before you serve it.

4.53 GRAVY

Cooking time: 20 minutes

Ingredients

- 1quart chicken stock
- 2 onions, diced
- 2 garlic cloves
- pan drippings
- 1/2 teaspoon salt
- 1 tablespoon thyme, minced

Instructions

1. Bring chicken stock, onions, and garlic to a boil in a medium saucepan. Reduce heat to low and cook for 30 minutes, or until onions and garlic are tender. Pour the drippings from the pan into a saucepan. Using an immersion blender or a blender, puree the stock-onion-drippings combination. Reheat the mixture in the pot, then season with salt and thyme. Serve with turkey, mashed cauliflower, or as dressing.

4.54 Tahini Sauce

Cooking time: 5 minutes

Ingredients

- 1/4 cup warm water
- 1/3 cup tahini
- 1 teaspoon orange zest
- 1 teaspoon fresh lemon juice
- 1 tablespoon cilantro leaves, diced
- 1 tablespoon tamari

Instructions

1. Whisk together all of the ingredients in a medium mixing basin. You can add more water if you want a thinner sauce. And it is ready to serve.

4.55 Turkey Burger

Cooking time: 25 minutes

Ingredients

- 1 lb. turkey
- 1/4 cup onion, diced
- 1/4 teaspoon diced garlic
- 1 tablespoon tamari
- 2 tablespoons flour
- 3 tablespoons parmesan
- 2 tablespoons mayonnaise
- salt and pepper

Instructions

1. Make flat patties using the mixture. 2 tablespoons olive oil in a nonstick pan Cook for 2 minutes on medium-high after searing/browning the first side. Reduce heat to low, turn, and cook for another 2 to 3 minutes. Top with a thin coating of miso and a sprinkling of grated parmesan cheese.

4.56 Fruit Sorbet

Cooking time: 20 minutes

Ingredients

- 2 bananas
- 1 cup strawberries
- 2 tablespoons water
- 1 tablespoon lemon juice

Instructions

1. Bananas should be peeled and sliced into 1-inch pieces. Place the bananas and strawberries on a rimmed baking sheet coated with wax paper. Freeze until solid. In a food processor, puree the fruit, water, and lemon juice until smooth. Serve right away or freeze for up to two weeks. Serve with whole strawberries as a garnish.

4.57 Vegan Ice Cream

Cooking time: 10 minutes

Ingredients

- 2 cups water
- 1 cup diced cashews
- honey
- 2 cups fruit of choice (mango, peaches)

Instructions

1. Blend cashews in a food processor to produce a fine meal (about 3-4 minutes). After that, add water and honey to taste. Add the fruit and process until the cashews are no longer gritty. Chill for 15 minutes in the freezer before pouring into an ice cream machine. Process them for about half an hour and serve them immediately.

4.58 Peanut Sauce

Cooking time: 10 minutes

Ingredients

- 1/4 cup peanut butter
- 1/4 cup coconut milk
- 2 tablespoons lime juice
- 1 tablespoon tamari
- 2 teaspoons honey
- 1/2 tablespoon red pepper

Instructions

1. In a big mixing bowl, combine all of the ingredients. Whisk everything together until it is fully smooth and then it is ready to serve.

4.59 MEATBALLS

Cooking time: 30 minutes

Ingredients

- 2 pounds ground turkey
- 1 egg
- 3/4 cup non-dairy cheese
- 1/2 cup flour
- 2 garlic cloves
- 1 teaspoon oregano
- 1/2 teaspoon rosemary
- 1/2 teaspoon basil
- 1/2 teaspoon salt
- pinch of pepper

Instructions

1. To avoid overworking, combine everything using a big fork. (Meatballs that have been overworked will be thick.) Before making meatballs, run your hands under cold water. In comparison to beef meatballs, they'll be a little sticky. Make big meatballs. Bake for 45 minutes at 350 degrees on a sheet pan.

4.60 BISCUITS

Cooking time: 25 minutes

Ingredients

- 2 cups flour

- 1/2 teaspoon salt

- 1/2 teaspoon baking soda

- 1/4 cup oil

- 1/4 cup honey

- 2 eggs

- 1 teaspoon lemon juice

Instructions

1. Preheat the oven to 350 degrees Fahrenheit. Using parchment paper, line a large baking sheet. Combine the almond flour, salt, and baking soda in a large mixing basin. Whisk together the canola oil, honey, eggs, and lemon juice in a medium mixing bowl. Combine the wet components and stir them into the almond flour mixture until everything is well mixed. Drop the batter onto the baking sheet in scant 14 cup increments, 2 inches apart. Bake until golden brown or a toothpick inserted in the center of a biscuit comes out clean, 15 to 20 minutes. Allow the biscuits to cool on the baking sheet for a few minutes before serving warm.

4.61 BEAN SOUP

Cooking time: 15 minutes

Ingredients

- 2 tablespoon oil
- 1 can of beans, cooked
- 1 onion
- 1/2 cup carrots, chopped
- 1/2 cup celery
- 8 cups vegetable broth
- 1 can tomatoes
- 1 can tomato sauce
- 1 garlic clove
- 3 cups kale
- 1 teaspoon oregano
- 1 teaspoon rosemary
- Salt and pepper to taste

Instructions

1. Heat the oil in a big saucepan. Start frying the carrots, celery, and onions when it shimmers, and simmer until the onions are transparent. Combine the beans, vegetable broth, tomatoes, tomato sauce, barley, garlic, and spices in a large mixing bowl. Bring to a boil, then lower to low heat and cook for 1 hour. Remove the lid and simmer for another 30 minutes, adding the kale in the last 10 minutes of cooking.

4.62 Fruit Salad Smoothie

Cooking time: 5 minutes

Ingredients

- 1 cup fresh orange juice
- 1 banana
- 1/2 cup mango, peaches
- 1 cup plant-based yogurt
- few ice cubes

Instructions

1. Fill a blender halfway with juice. Blend in the fruit and yogurt until smooth. Towards the ending of the mixing process, add the ice.

4.63 Fruit Sauce

Cooking time: 15 minutes

Ingredients

- 1 pear
- 1 kiwi
- 2 nectarines
- 2 apricots
- 1 chili pepper
- 1/2 cup diced onions
- 1 avocado
- 1/2 cup diced cilantro
- 1/2 cup lime juice

Instructions

1. Cut the nectarines, pear, and apricots into tiny pieces after removing the seeds. Peel the kiwi and proceed in the same manner. In a large mixing basin, combine all of the fruit. Remove the seeds from the chili and cut them into very small pieces. Toss the onion and chili into the fruit bowl. Cut the avocado in half, scoop out the flesh, and toss it in with the other ingredients. Combine the chopped cilantro and the lime juice in a mixing bowl. Mix all of the ingredients together until they are well combined. Serve right away.

4.64 Melon Pops

Cooking time: 15 minutes

Ingredients

- 6ounces orange juice (frozen)
- 1/2 chopped cantaloupe
- 1 cup non-dairy yogurt
- 1 cup berries (if tolerated)
- 1 ripe banana

Instructions

1. In a blender or food processor, combine all of the ingredients and mix until smooth. On a tray, arrange about 15 3 oz. paper cups for freezing. Fill cups 3/4 full with the mixture. Using a knife, cut a tiny slit in the center of each cup's foil. In the slit, place the popsicle stick upright.

4.65 Salmon Patties

Cooking time: 20 minutes

Ingredients

- 1 can salmon
- 1 egg
- 1/2 cup breadcrumbs
- 1 tablespoon oil

Instructions

1. In a mixing dish, combine all of the ingredients. Form patties from the mixture. Cook for several minutes on each side in a skillet over medium heat until browned.

4.66 Easy Vegetable Mash

Cooking time: 10 minutes

Ingredients

- 2pound root veggies
- 1/2 cup bone broth
- 2 tablespoon oil
- 1 teaspoon salt
- pinch of black pepper

Instructions

1. Cook or steam the vegetables until they are extremely soft, then mash them well. Stir in the broth, oil, salt, and pepper to the vegetables.

4.67 Rice Noodles With Tofu

Cooking time: 25 minutes

Ingredients

- 1 tablespoon oil
- 1 tablespoon peanut butter
- 1 tablespoon maple syrup
- 3 tablespoons soy sauce
- 2 tablespoons lemon juice
- 1 block tofu
- 2 cups frozen veggies
- 1 can corn
- 6 oz. rice noodles
- Cilantro

Instructions

1. Preheat the oven to 400 degrees Fahrenheit. Tofu should be cut into cubes. Toss the tofu with the first five ingredients that have been whisked together. Bake the tofu for 20 to 25 minutes on a prepared baking sheet. Cook rice noodles as directed on the box. In a large skillet, heat 2 tablespoons of sesame oil and sauté veggies until soft. To serve, divide the noodles into two bowls and top with the vegetables, tofu, and cilantro.

4.68 FRUIT MUFFINS

Cooking time: 30 minutes

Ingredients

- 1/2 cup flour
- 1/2 cup brown sugar
- 1/2 teaspoon salt
- 2 tablespoons baking powder
- 3 tablespoons melted butter
- 1 cup of non-dairy milk
- 1 egg
- 1 teaspoon vanilla extract
- 1 cup of frozen fruit

Instructions

1. Preheat the oven to 375 degrees Fahrenheit. Set aside the muffin cups after greasing them. Set aside a bowl containing the flour, sugar, salt, and baking powder. Combine the melted butter or oil, egg, and vanilla essence in a separate dish. Combine all the wet and dry ingredients in a mixing bowl. Fill the muffin cups halfway with the frozen fruits, then bake for 25 minutes.

4.69 Tuna With Noodles

Cooking time: 25 minutes

Ingredients

- 8 oz. noodles
- 1 bag snow peas
- 1/4 cup soy sauce
- 2 tablespoons lime juice
- 2 tablespoons oil
- 1/4 cup cilantro leaves
- 4 tablespoons sesame seeds
- 2 tuna steaks
- cooking spray
- 1/2 teaspoon salt
- 1 tablespoon oil

Instructions

1. Cook the noodles as directed on the box. During the last 3 minutes of cooking, add the snow peas. Drain thoroughly after rinsing with warm water. In a large mixing bowl, whisk together the soy sauce, lime juice, chili sauce, and sesame oil. Toss in the noodles and cilantro to incorporate. In a shallow plate, combine white and black sesame seeds. Spray the tuna steaks with cooking spray and season with salt equally. Sprinkle sesame seeds on both sides of each steak and gently press to adhere. In a big skillet, heat the vegetable oil over medium-high heat. Cook for 3 minutes on each side for medium-rare tuna, or until desired.

4.70 Sushi

Cooking time: 25 minutes

Ingredients

- 1 Sushi packet
- 5 tablespoons mayonnaise
- 1 avocado
- 250g Salmon (smoked)
- 1 carrot
- 1/2 teaspoon wasabi
- 2 cups sushi rice

Instructions

1. Cook the rice according to the package directions. Cut the carrot, avocado into thin strips while the rice is cooking. Combine the mayonnaise and wasabi in a mixing bowl. Allow for some cooling time once the rice has been cooked before beginning to form your rolls. Using a knife, cut a sheet of sushi in two. Spread a little amount of mayonnaise diagonally over the sheet from the top left corner to the middle bottom. Add a strip of rice on top of it, then a slice of smoked salmon, and finally your veggies. Enjoy by rolling the sushi into a cone shape.

4.71 Veggie Frittata

Cooking time: 15 minutes

Ingredients

- veggies combination
- 3 eggs
- 1 teaspoon salt
- a pinch of black pepper
- 1 teaspoon oregano

Instructions

1. Preheat the oven to 180 degrees Celsius (350F). In a mixing bowl, whisk together the three eggs, add the herbs, salt, and pepper, and then pour the mixture into an oven-safe dish (make sure the dish is non-stick, or oil/line it with greaseproof paper first to prevent your frittata from sticking to the bottom of the pan). Make sure the eggs are thick enough to cover the bottom of the pan, about 1-2cm thick. Prepare your veggies by slicing them thinly and placing them in the egg mixture. You have to preheat the oven to 350°F and bake for 30 minutes. When the frittata is done, it should have a golden brown color to it.

4.72 Samphire With Sesame Oil

Cooking time: 10 minutes

Ingredients

- 2 cups samphire
- sesame oil

Instructions

- In a large frying pan, heat the sesame oil over medium heat. Add the samphire and cook for a couple minutes, while stirring regularly. Add seasoning by taste.

4.73 Omelette

Cooking time: 10 minutes

Ingredients

- 2 eggs
- non-dairy cheese
- 1/2 cup mushrooms
- 1/2 cup peppers
- 1 teaspoon zucchini
- 1 teaspoon olive oil
- salt and pepper to taste

Instructions

1. In a mixing dish, crack the eggs and whisk them together. Heat the oil in a frying pan. Add all of the ingredients to the pan, except the egg and cheese, and soften them for a few minutes. Slightly, remove the pan from the heat and set it aside. Allow the eggs to spread out before adding them. For a minute, cook. Only one side of the eggs should have all the cooked ingredients and the cheese. Fold the egg over on itself and heat for another minute or until the cheese has melted. Remove the pan from the heat and it is ready to serve.

4.74 Spaghetti Bolognese

Cooking time: 25 minutes

Ingredients

- 200g spaghetti
- 1 can tomato puree
- 2 tablespoons olive oil
- 1 garlic clove
- 1/2 onion
- 1 teaspoon rosemary
- 200g beef mince

Instructions

1. In a heavy-bottomed pan, heat the oil and sauté the garlic, onion, rosemary, and bacon until softened for about 5 minutes. Break up the beef mince with your fingers as you put it into the pan. Cook, stirring occasionally, for a few minutes, until the mince begins to brown. Break up the tomatoes in the pan and add them. Allow simmering for about 45 minutes, covered. If it becomes too dry, a little water can be added. Meanwhile, boil the pasta according to the package directions and serve immediately with the sauce.

4.75 Non-Dairy Custard

Cooking time: 10 minutes

Ingredients

- 2 egg yolks
- 1 teaspoon brown sugar
- 1/4 teaspoon vanilla extract
- 1 teaspoon corn flour
- 1 cup almond milk

Instructions

1. In a mixing dish, combine the yolk, sugar, and corn flour. Bring the milk and vanilla extract to a low boil in a saucepan. Return to the fire and stir until the custard has thickened, then pour the milk over the egg mixture.

4.76 Summer Salad

Cooking time: 10 minutes

Ingredients

- 1 apple, diced
- 2 carrots, diced
- 1/4 cup lemon juice
- 1 tablespoon non-dairy yogurt
- 1/4 tablespoon honey
- 1 tablespoon sesame seeds

Instructions

1. In a mixing dish, combine the grated apple, carrots, and lemon juice. Combine the yogurt and honey in a separate bowl. Stir the two together thoroughly. Sesame seeds should be sprinkled on top.

4.77 Basil Courgettes

Cooking time: 20 minutes

Ingredients

- 1 diced courgette
- 1 tablespoon olive oil
- 1/2 tablespoon lemon juice
- 1 tablespoon basil
- salt and pepper to taste

Instructions

1. Heat the oil in a frying pan. Place the courgettes in the pan one by one, in a single layer. Cook for a few minutes on one side and then flip and do the same on the other side. Remove the pan from the heat and stir in the lemon juice, black pepper, and torn basil.

4.78 Minty Tabbouleh

Cooking time: 15 minutes

Ingredients

- 1 cup quinoa
- 2 chopped chives
- 2 teaspoons diced mint leaves
- 1 teaspoon diced parsley
- 2 tablespoons olive oil
- 2 tablespoons lime juice

Instructions

1. Cook the quinoa as directed on the package. Add the herbs and the lemon juice. Season with salt to taste. Stir for 10 minutes and then it is ready to serve.

4.79 ORANGE TRUFFLES

Cooking time: 25 minutes

Ingredients

- 1 cup pecans
- 2 cups dates
- 1 orange (zest)
- 2 tablespoons maple syrup
- 2 tablespoons powdered cocoa

Instructions

1. Blend the pecan nuts in a food processor until they are fine crumbs. Blend in the dates until they are all broken up and evenly distributed throughout the nuts. Blend together the cocoa powder, maple syrup, and orange zest. If the mixture clings to the side, use a knife to loosen it and blend it again. Roll the mixture into bite-size pieces, then coat with additional cocoa powder or pecan nuts. You will finish up with about 15-20 balls. Allow chilling for a few minutes before serving.

4.80 Grapefruit Sorbet

Cooking time: 30 minutes

Ingredients

- 1 1/2 cups brown sugar

- 1 3/4 water

- 1 cup grapefruit juice

- 1/4 lemon juice

- 1 egg white

- 1 tablespoon grapefruit zest

Instructions

1. Combine the sugar, grapefruit zest, and water in a mixing bowl. Bring the water to a boil. When the sugar is melted right, remove it from the heat. Lemon juice and pink grapefruit juice are added. Refrigerate for six hours after transferring the sorbet mix to a storage container. Mix in the barely beaten egg white until everything is well combined. In an ice cream maker, freeze the sorbet mixture according to the manufacturer's guidelines. Place the sorbet in a freezer-safe container and freeze for 2 hours before serving.

4.81 Lemon Tart

Cooking time: 30 minutes

Ingredients

- 1 cup flour
- 5 tablespoons vegetable shortening
- 1 cup brown sugar
- 2 tablespoons flour
- 2 teaspoons lemon zest
- 1/2 teaspoon baking powder
- 2 eggs
- pinch of salt
- 1/2 cup lemon juice

Instructions

1. Combine 1 cup flour, sugar, and vegetable shortening until a coarse meal is formed. In a lightly oiled baking dish, press the mixture into the bottom. As usual, preheat the oven to 350°F and bake for 20 minutes. Incorporate the remaining ingredients in a separate bowl and stir to combine. Pour them over the crust that has been cooked. Cook for another 20 to 25 minutes in the oven. It's ready after 30 minutes of cooling.

4.82 date banana smoothie

Cooking time: 5 minutes

Ingredients

- 1 cup almond milk
- 2 packed cups kale leaves
- 2 teaspoons lemon juice
- 1/2 cup diced dates
- 1 sliced banana

Instructions

1. Add the almond milk, kale, and lemon juice; pulse to break up the greens, then mix for 20 seconds to 1 minute. Blend in the dates and banana until the mixture is thick enough.

4.83 Coriander Soup

Cooking time: 25 minutes

Ingredients

- 1 onion
- 1 pound of carrots
- 1 bunch cilantro
- 1 tablespoon oil
- 1 tablespoon coriander
- 2pints vegetable stock

Instructions

1. In a large pan, heat the oil and add the onions and carrots. Cook for 10-15 minutes, covered. Season with salt and pepper after adding the ground coriander. Bring the stock to a boil, then remove from the heat. Reduce the heat to low and continue to cook until the veggies are soft. Blend until smooth, either with an immersion blender or in a blender. Reheat in a clean pan, then serve with fresh cilantro on top.

4.84 Mango Salsa

Cooking time: 10 minutes

Ingredients

- 2 mangoes
- 1 serrano chili pepper
- 2 onions
- 1/2 red pepper
- 1/2 yellow pepper
- 1 cup chopped cilantro
- 1 juiced lime

Instructions

1. In a dish, combine the mango pieces. Add the chopped chili pepper, spring onions, red and yellow bell peppers, and salt and pepper to taste. Combine the cilantro and lime juice in a mixing bowl. If required, add extra lime juice. Allow 1 hour before serving in the refrigerator.

4.85 Spinach Dip

Cooking time: 10 minutes

Ingredients

- 1 can artichoke
- 1 package frozen spinach
- 1 cup non-dairy yogurt
- 1 cup non-dairy cheese
- 1 garlic clove
- 2 tablespoons red pepper

Instructions

1. Mix all of the ingredients, except the red pepper, well. Fill a plate halfway with the mixture. Sprinkle with red peppers and bake at 350 degrees for 20-25 minutes, or until cooked through. Serve alongside vegetables.

4.86 Kale Chips

Cooking time: 25 minutes

Ingredients

- 1 bunch kale
- 1 tablespoon olive oil
- salt, pepper

Instructions

1. Preheat oven to 350 degrees. Using parchment paper, line a cookie sheet. Remove the leaves off the thick stems of kale with a knife or kitchen shears and shred them into bite-size pieces. Using a salad spinner, thoroughly dry the kale. Drizzle kale with olive oil and season with salt and pepper to taste. Bake the chips for 10 - 15 minutes, or until the edges are brown but not burned.

4.87 Bean Dip

Cooking time: 10 minutes

Ingredients

- 1 can beans
- 1 garlic clove
- 2 tablespoons lime juice
- 2 tablespoons olive oil
- 1/4 cup parsley leaves
- salt and pepper

Instructions

1. Combine all ingredients in a blender. Blend until it is smooth and it is ready to serve.

4.88 Stuffed Mushrooms

Cooking time: 30 minutes

Ingredients

- 1 pound of mushrooms
- 4 oz. diced spinach
- 3 oz. vegan cheese
- 3 garlic cloves
- 1 egg
- 1/4 cup parmesan
- salt

Instructions

1. Preheat oven to 400 degrees. Remove stems and clean mushrooms with a dry brush or cloth. Chop the stems and mix them with the rest of the ingredients. Place mushroom caps on a baking sheet and pour the mixture into each cap from the bowl. You should bake the dish for 15 minutes on the top rack of the oven.

4.89 Green Beans

Cooking time: 30 minutes

Ingredients

- 1 pound green beans
- 1 onion
- 3 garlic cloves
- 1 tablespoon oil
- 1 teaspoon paprika
- 1 can tomatoes

Instructions

1. Green beans should be steamed for 5 minutes before being rapidly chilled in cold water. Remove from the equation. 3 minutes in a medium skillet, sauté onion and garlic in oil. Add the paprika and the tomato juice you set aside. Cook, stirring constantly until the liquid has thickened somewhat. Mix in the tomatoes and green beans that were set aside. Cook, stirring constantly, for 2 minutes over medium heat, or until cooked through and beans are tender-crisp.

4.90 SANDWICH BREAD

Cooking time: 60 minutes

Ingredients

- 3/4 cup almond butter
- 4 eggs
- 1 cup flour
- 1 teaspoon salt
- 1 teaspoon baking soda
- 1 tablespoon flax meal

Instructions

1. Preheat oven to 350 degrees. The oil and almond flour are used to grease a loaf pan. Mix the almond butter and eggs together in another dish until smooth. Combine the almond flour, salt, baking soda, and flax meal. Combine the almond flour and wet ingredients in a blender and blend until smooth. Fill the loaf pan halfway with batter. Bake on the bottom rack of the oven for 40 to 45 minutes, or until a knife inserted in the center comes out clean. Allow one hour for the bread to cool in the pan before serving.

4.91 CHUTNEY

Ingredients

- 1pound tart apples
- 1 bag of cranberries
- 1 cup honey
- 1 cup vinegar
- 1 tablespoon cinnamon
- 1 tablespoon ginger
- 1 teaspoon red pepper flakes
- 1/2 pound raisins

Instructions

1. Combine all ingredients in a large saucepan and cook for about 30 minutes. You can taste to know if it is done. Let it cool off and it is ready to serve.

4.92 Ketchup

Cooking time: 15 minutes

Ingredients

- 12 oz. tomato puree
- 4 tablespoons vinegar
- 1 tablespoon mustard
- 1/2 cup water
- 1/2 teaspoon salt
- 1/2 teaspoon cinnamon
- 1/8 teaspoon garlic powder

Instructions

1. Whisk together all of the ingredients. You may want to combine the spices to ensure that they are uniformly distributed. It's ideal to leave the ketchup in the fridge for a few hours or overnight to allow the flavors to meld properly.

4.93 Tuna Salad

Cooking time: 10 minutes

Ingredients

- 2 cans tuna
- 1 can beans
- 10 cherry tomatoes
- 4 green onions
- 1 tablespoon olive oil
- 1 tablespoon lemon juice
- salt and pepper

Instructions

1. In a medium mixing bowl, combine tuna, drained beans, tomatoes, scallions, olive oil, lemon juice, and pepper. Gently stir the ingredients together. Place in the refrigerator to cool off until ready to serve.

4.94 Nutty Smoothie

Cooking time: 5 minutes

Ingredients

- 1/2 cup soy milk
- 1/2 cup non-dairy yogurt
- 1 tablespoon honey
- 1/3 cup almond butter
- 2 bananas

Instructions

1. Mix all the ingredients into a blender. Blend until smooth and serve.

4.95 Medallions

Cooking time: 20 minutes

Ingredients

- 2pounds turkey tenderloin
- 1 tablespoon olive oil
- 2 garlic cloves
- 3 shallots
- 1 cup diced apple
- 1/2 cup orange juice

Instructions

1. Place the turkey tenderloins in a baking dish that has been gently oiled. Apply a light layer of olive oil to the surface. In a saucepan, combine the remaining ingredients and bring to a boil. Reduce the heat to low, so it does not burn, and cook for 5 minutes. Pour the sauce over the turkey. Bake for 1 hour or until done, uncovered, at 350°F.

4.96 Butter Rolls

Cooking time: 10 minutes

Ingredients

- 2 bananas
- 1/4 cup butter
- 1/4 cup chocolate shavings

Instructions

1. Each banana should be cut into four segments. Spread some butter on each of the banana slices using a knife. Fill a dish with chocolate shavings. Each banana should be rolled in the shavings. The chocolate shavings will stick to the melted butter.

4.97 Chicken Strips

Cooking time: 15 minutes

Ingredients

- 1.5pound skinless chicken breast
- 2 tablespoons lemon juice
- 2 garlic cloves
- 3 tablespoons olive oil
- 2 tablespoons diced parsley
- salt and pepper

Instructions

1. In a zip lock bag, combine lemon juice, garlic, olive oil, pepper, and parsley to make a marinade for chicken. Add the chicken and marinate for at least 1 hour in the refrigerator. Cook until tender and white through on the grill or on the stovetop.

4.98 Pizza

Cooking time: 40 minutes

Ingredients

- 2 tablespoons oil
- 2 cups flour
- 2 eggs
- 1/2 cup vegan cheese
- 1/4 teaspoon salt
- 2 cups tomato sauce
- 1 teaspoon oregano
- 1/2 cup non-dairy cheese

Instructions

1. Preheat the oven to 350 degrees. Set aside a baking dish or a circular pizza pan greased with a teaspoon of canola oil. To prepare the crust, whisk together the olive oil, almond flour, eggs, farmer's cheese, and salt in a mixing bowl. Roll it into a ball and place it in a greased baking dish, patting it down to form a thin layer. Preheat the oven to 200°F and bake for 20 minutes, or until golden brown. Remove the pizza from the oven and cover it with tomato sauce, oregano, and low-fat cheese. Return the casserole to the oven for a further 5 minutes, or until the cheese has melted.

4.99 LASAGNA

Cooking time: 45 minutes

Ingredients

- 2 zucchini
- 1 cup tomato sauce
- 1/4 cup olive oil
- 1/2 cup non-dairy cheese
- 1/2 cup parmesan

Instructions

1. Preheat oven to 375 degrees. Cut the zucchini lengthwise into long, thin slices using a sharp knife. Fill a baking dish with 1/3 cup tomato sauce. Drizzle olive oil over one-third of the zucchini. One-third of each of the cheeses should be sprinkled on top. Rep the procedure, adding two more layers each time, until all of the components have been used. Bake for 40 to 45 minutes, or until bubbling on top, uncovered in the oven. Allow the dish to cool off for a few minutes before slicing.

4.100 Tofu With Almond Sauce

Cooking time: 30 minutes

Ingredients

- 2 tablespoons vinegar

- 1 tablespoon tamari

- 1 package of tofu

- 1/2 cup almond butter

- 1 cup soy milk

- 1 garlic clove

- 2 tablespoons ginger

- 1 tablespoon sesame oil

- 1 onion

- salt and pepper

Instructions

1. Combine the vinegar and tamari in a large mixing dish. Toss the cubed tofu in the marinade and toss to coat. Combine all of the ingredients in a blender, or maybe a food processor if you have, and purée the ingredients until they are smooth. Put the ingredients in a frying pan and cook for 10-15 minutes. Let it cool off and it is ready to serve.

Conclusion

Every patient with Ulcerative Colitis must take an active role in their therapy. They should be aware of the extent of their illness, the drugs they've taken, what has helped and what hasn't, as well as whether or not they've experienced any adverse effects and what they were. Because Ulcerative Colitis is a chronic condition that will affect you for the rest of your life, you should choose the proper healthcare expert to assist you in effectively manage your illness.

If the treatment that you are already practicing is not providing you good results, you should tell your doctor. Both you and your healthcare expert can work on the perfect diet plan and medication treatment for your Ulcerative Colitis condition. Keeping a food journal will help you discover which food triggers your symptoms and which is good for you. This is also important since you will know how to avoid a flare-up by not eating or drinking anything you already know might provoke symptoms. You may be able to consume a wide variety of foods until you get a flare-up. However, you, like everyone else, must make good food choices. However, even the healthiest meals might aggravate symptoms. It may be beneficial to keep note of your "problem foods." Any queries you have regarding healthy eating should be directed to your healthcare professional.

As someone suffering from Ulcerative Colitis, being your own advocate is one of the most essential things you can do for yourself. When speaking with your doctors, do not be afraid to express yourself. Ask as many questions as you want, and be open about your feelings regarding the treatment you are receiving. Ulcerative Colitis may be very difficult on your stomach, and you may need to change your diet during a flare-up, possibly sticking to a BRAT diet, which contains banana, rice, applesauce, and toast. So, when you enter remission, you might be allowed to celebrate by eating foods that bring you joy and taste great. You should, however, be careful and try to avoid aggravating your symptoms unintentionally.

Even if you have Ulcerative Colitis, you can live a full life. Concentrate on maintaining control over your symptoms. Also, do not let the illness isolate you. You can deal by planning ahead of time and engaging with support groups. You might even be able to assist those who suffer from Ulcerative Colitis.

You should practice eating more small meals rather than three large meals, especially if you are on the road or you do not have quick access to a restroom. If you have just experienced a flare-up, consume items that you know will help you manage your symptoms. Both at home and at work, have those meals on hand. Discuss your plans with your healthcare advisor if you are planning a long trip. If you suffer a flare-up while driving or being on the road, he or she can advise you on what to do. And this can help you manage your symptoms and feel better. Living with the disease can be really hard that is why it is important for you to learn about it and how to manage it.

"With that in mind, we would like to thank you for choosing this book as a guide to help you combat Ulcerative Colitis. We would also like to ask you to take some time to give the book a positive rating, as it will help other people who are suffering from the same disease find it and make their lives easier and healthier."

Printed in Great Britain
by Amazon